Seemingly Sound Eating yet

SEVERE
BODILY DAMAGE

Inflammation Is Silently Assassinating You

ROBIN DOBBINS

authorHOUSE®

AuthorHouse™
1663 Liberty Drive
Bloomington, IN 47403
www.authorhouse.com
Phone: 1 (800) 839-8640

Published by AuthorHouse 11/16/2015

ISBN: 978-1-5049-5794-6 (sc)
ISBN: 978-1-5049-5793-9 (e)

Library of Congress Control Number: 2015917607

Print information available on the last page.

Any people depicted in stock imagery provided by Thinkstock are models, and such images are being used for illustrative purposes only. Certain stock imagery © Thinkstock.

This book is printed on acid-free paper.

Because of the dynamic nature of the Internet, any web addresses or links contained in this book may have changed since publication and may no longer be valid. The views expressed in this work are solely those of the author and do not necessarily reflect the views of the publisher, and the publisher hereby disclaims any responsibility for them.

Table of Contents

Foreword

Through some unexpected circumstances, which will later be explained, I am a practicing certified personal fitness trainer (CPFT) and rehabilitative exercise specialist (RES) for hire, working out of a community fitness center in LaPorte, Texas. This unique city, of approximately 34,000 people, lies just southeast of Houston. During the 15 years at this facility, age ranges of my "victims" has varied from an eight year-old figure skater to a 93 year-old with Alzheimer's. I have, however, developed a niche for those old enough to qualify for Social Security. This is a segment of our nation's population being left behind in the health and fitness industry; maybe "given-up on" or ignored is a better description. Although getting stronger is their main need, eating too, like the much more emphasized portion of the population, is a real concern. It's here, I found the inspiration to write this book. I'm doing it for those old enough to be afraid – scared of eating in a manner that causes life's real ailments to worsen. There are certainly more serious considerations than being overweight.

Jack LaLane once said, he exercised and ate healthy in order "...to live while living." At age 15, Jack was told his eating like a human garbage can had left him in deplorable health. Shortly afterward, the youngster got down on his knees and prayed, "God give me the strength to stay away from all that junk food that is killing me." From then on, Jack screamed, "I was born again!" The rest of his life was nothing short of legendary on the health and fitness scales. He died in 2011 at age 96.

Fortunately, I was privileged to spend two weeks with this guru of fitness back in 1969 or '70; my memory is waning. His palatial gym in Oakland, California was the scene of some awesome instruction and fun times. The man was about 5'5" or so in height and looked to weigh 160-170 pounds; no fat. This guy worked out (weights) with speed and intensity such as no one was accustomed. So much so, I had to use a much lighter weight to perform the exercises. The "humbling" adjustment did not prevent my becoming oxygen deficient enough to avoid making an embarrassing run to the locker room for the purpose of "upchucking." At the time, we had been working those huge back muscles, which require more oxygen than any other muscle group, with the exception of legs. It was not uncommon back then to "vomit" on leg day during the cut-up phase preparing for a bodybuilding contest. During my tutelage with the man, he knew I had been in the building up phase – size and strength. Lifting heavy weights with low reps and appropriate rest between sets was my routine; oxygen deficiency was not going to happen. Many big name Spartans of the black iron had turned down Jack's invitation to participate in his routine. The list was a very distinguished one at that.

Before my brief stint with LaLane, I was training under the watchful eye of Jack Delinger, Mr. Universe 1956. One day he put one of those big arms over my shoulder and informed me of an arrangement he made with Mr. LaLane to further my schooling. Upon returning two weeks later, he asked how my diet of humility tasted. I realized Mr. Delinger felt some fatherly responsibility in my "upbringing." The lesson learned.

For both guys, eating was simple; don't accept anything from a box – no processed foods. That was actually swell advice back then, considering not much science had entered the picture. Very little consideration was given to cholesterol (clogged arteries), and inflammation was not even a gleam in "his" daddy's eyes. For the reason of my height and desire to compete in bodybuilding and powerlifting back then, I was placed on what amounted to a 10,000 calorie per day diet from Parillo. It was very difficult to abandon that plan, when necessary, as evidenced by my triple by-pass in November of 2012. Went in for a heart valve replacement (pig valve), and the surgeon discovered three arteries had blockages of 70, 40, and 60 percent. The bad heart valve had been standard equipment, when I was born.

Quarts of half and half to go along with consuming an occasional 2 lb. Velveeta cheese bar at one sitting sufficed as snacks. For your information, a quart of half & half contains 32 servings. Did you get that? For me, the quart had but one serving. From recollection, the cheese bar rendered a whopping 2,400 calories, 94 grams of protein, and 96 grams of fat. A protein drink consisted of dropping a dozen eggs in a blender filled with whipped cream. For flavor, a pint of Lady Borden ice cream was squeezed in with two scoops of chalk flavored protein, whose trade name was Incal. Blend that up and tell me it doesn't taste great! Arteries would have been plugged much sooner had not the rest of my food intake been impeccable. Aside from the cheese bar and ice cream, all foods I consumed were considered healthy choices; "good ole boys".

A famous Mr. Olympia, I was fortunate enough to work with while in California, had me try still another experiment. What a joyful surprise! It entailed restricting my meat of choice to beef; four pounds per day for an entire month. There was a God after all. Four pounds of porterhouse steaks every day was a dream! I got noticeably bigger and stronger; felt great with energy off-the-chart. The next month meat was restricted to anything but beef. Please no! I remember tuna was nine cents a can, and chicken too was a giveaway. My wife, Janel, bless her wonderful heart, loved the lower grocery tab, but this body hated the results; lost weight, strength, and energy. You see, beef naturally contains creatine, one of today's prime supplements for power athletes. I won't bore you with its dynamic workings.

Ross Querry (PT, Ph.D.), a renowned dietician and muscle science genius (among other things), recommends eating chicken and supplementing creatine. I have since taken his advice to heart; for the most part. He is a very impressive force in an industry with much "bologna." Met the man at a workshop entitled: "Power in Motion."

During the fall of 2000, while working as an operations technician at Lyondell-Basell (a major world player in the chemical industry), one fitness manager for a major health club chain asked if I would help train the trainers at his locale (part-time), in addition to working with some assigned members. A week or so prior, another gentleman, who owned a nutrition store (Supplement Depot), had asked if I would manage a fitness center he was planning to establish on site; choose my hours. Both offers were intriguing, but I leaned toward managing the fitness center and retiring from shift work. For various reasons the center failed to materialize, so I accepted the position at the health club. Didn't much care for instructing the "inexperienced know-it-all" trainers, but surprisingly found helping those unfamiliar with "black iron" rather rewarding.

At this point, obtaining a personal fitness trainer certificate became imperative, just in case I decided someday to "lite-out" on my own. After all, the day of written credentials and documentation had arrived. The chosen program was run by an organization for Baylor Sports Medicine Institute named PFIT (Personal Fitness Instructor Training). The manual itself was 3" thick (giant three-ring binder), and the course was five nights a week, plus half day on Saturday for thirteen weeks. The test consisted of 500 written questions, followed by a three-hour practicum. Pressure was such that many did not even complete the written exam while others left the practicum room before finishing. Something like 127 signed up, and a mere 47 or so passed.

A few months later, I was invited to attempt the Rehabilitative Exercise Specialist certification. Through the grace of God, I managed to succeed. The format was the same as the CPFT, but the total success number was considerably lower. Being capable of rehabilitating someone who had surgery proved rewarding. I usually take them after their insurance ceases to pay a rehab center. It has been my good fortune to help people avoid surgery, and many times perform the rehab continuum from the beginning. There are no words for this wonderful experience.

PFIT is owned by two overqualified and wonderful people; Wayne and Dahelia Hunt. Their required continuing education workshops and seminars are quality and fun off-the-chart. The Hunts may be contacted at PFIT.org. Andy Cox taught the RES certification for the most part, and continued to help me well after my obtaining the certification. He is a caring, awesome fella. We have not had contact for a long while; back then, Andy was leading the Fondren Group; upscale rehab facilities.

Today, I endeavor 25-35 hours a week to make people physically stronger. The majority of my followers are over 60 years of age. The emphasis is on adding both muscle mass and bone density, while maintaining proper posture. You cannot separate the three. The object here is to keep them off a "walker" and allow daily activities to be easier. They want to be self-reliant for as long as possible. It's called a "quality life." There is little attention paid to us "old people." Most videos, magazines, etc., focus on the young "beautiful people."

Since realizing I really am old, it seems the industrial/technological societies wish we would just go away or accept the government's euthanasia package. Movies aren't made for us; cars aren't made for us; clothes aren't made for us, and crosswalks count off seconds now. We can't negotiate wide crosswalks in 12 seconds! Do we run back to the curb and start over or risk being flattened by a large SUV? Should the government round us up for disposal, think of all the jobs that'll be lost when oxygen bottles, walkers, and wheelchairs are no longer needed. So, I'm just trying to help "the living dead" (men and women) become capable of physically making it to the train headed for some place caring and appreciative of wisdom that only comes from living and living a long time. I don't know exactly where this tribal place may be, but it ain't here. Otherwise, we take our place in line for the Bataan Death March or Trail of Tears.

Eating correctly is as easy as two tablespoons of chocolate Ovaltine, secret code included. Don't let the beautiful people of this mega million dollar industry confuse you with complicated schemes. To give them their due, they are smart, research well, and have good intentions. But for you (myself included) geriatrics, or anyone else interested, drink your Ovaltine or read this children's book. Maybe both.

In the words of Alan Freed, "This is not good-bye; simply goodnight."

Signed,
Captain Midnight

> To be yourself in a world that is constantly
> trying to make you something else is
> the greatest accomplishment.
> -Ralph Waldo Emerson

Acknowledgments

I want to thank Janel Dobbins for her amazing perseverance, diligence, and skill in word processing this book from my hand-written hen-scratch. Each chapter had to be redone numerous times due to my mistakes and re-editing. I know there were times she just wanted this project to mercifully end; so did I. In case you didn't catch her last name, this wonderful woman is my wife and best friend.

I can't thank enough the authors of the following books and newsletters for their unbelievable research and knowledge. They inspired this meager attempt to make things simple for my clients and people like them.

Books & Hard Copy Newsletters
To My Home Mailbox

The Inflammation Free Diet Plan
    By Monica Reinagel
    Julius Torelli, M.D. (Consulting Editor)

The Blaylock Wellness Report (Hard copy to my home mailbox)
    By Dr. Russell Blaylock, Renowned Neurosurgeon
    Health Practitioner, Author, Lecturer

Ronald J. Grabowski, B.S., RD, DC
> Worldwide lecturer on nutritional health and founder of Innovative Nutritional Products.
>
> Attended two of his extraordinary seminars presented by Professional Fitness Instructor Training (PFIT). Sent three extremely overweight clients to him for dietary control and he worked wonders.

The Mind Health Report (Hard copy to my home mailbox)
> By Dr. Gary Small, Professor of Psychiatry & Aging
>> Director of UCLA Longevity Center

Trans Fat: The Hidden Killer In Our Food
> By Judith Shaw, M.A.

Toxic Relief
> By Don Colbert, M.D.

What You Don't Know May Be Killing You
> By Don Colbert, M.D.

Advanced Sports Nutrition
> By Dan Bernardot, Ph.D., RD, FACSM

Power Eating
> By Susan M. Kleiner, Ph.D., RD
> With Maggie Greenwood-Robinson

Eating on the Run
> By Evelyn Tribole, MS, RD

The Maker's Diet
> By Jordan S. Rubin
>> Foreword by Charles Stanley

The Carbohydrate Addict's Healthy Heart Program
     By Dr. Richard F. Heller
        Dr. Rachael F. Heller
        Dr. Frederic J. Vagnini

The Glucose Revolution
     By Helen O'Connor
        Jenner Brand-Miller, Ph.D.
        Stephen Colagiuri, M.D.
        Kay Foster-Powell, M.Nutr. & Diet
        Thomas M.S. Wolever, M.D. Ph.D.

Health Science Institute (Hard copy to my home mailbox)

E-Mail newsletters (countless articles):

Natural Health News & Self-Reliance
About Health: Tip of the Day
Doctor's House Call – Al Sears, M.D.
Life Script
BioTrust Nutrition
Life Enhancement
Dr. Whitaker newsletter

Introduction

There are 20,000 diet plans "out there" (i.e. Mediterranean, Paleo) and growing. Actually, several research groups put the number at 27,000. The Barnes & Noble bookstores have shelves upon shelves of books presenting these programs instructing us on eating correctly and combining foods properly. I have a cabinet filled with books on fitness and health; at least a dime's worth presenting diets and eating schemes alone. Many are designed to help one with the rather arduous task of keeping up with calories consumed and calories about to be consumed, while at the same time choosing foods that are truly nutritious. After all, it's highly possible to devour a bunch of "nutrition-empty" calories as your health eventually wanes. From there, the onslaught of publications covers carb counting, the glycemic index guide, diet cycling, fasting, juicing, "veganing," high-protein low-carb, and sundry of other topics. Ultimately, the emphasis is on changing the image of one's body composition from unfavorable to favorable through a sound eating and fitness regimen. **Wrong emphasis! These considerations will not help you avoid the silent but gradual erosion toward Alzheimer's, Parkinson's, heart disease, arthritis and an assortment of other crippling diseases that surface after age 50; ruining your "Golden Years." INFLAMMATION at the cellular level of both body and brain is the real felon, but yet is the least recognized or written about by mainstream health and fitness movers and shakers. It is without argument, amongst neurosurgeons and researchers alike, caused by the food we eat. If you eat to avoid inflammation, you'll not only avoid being disabled later in life, but your body composition will fall into place as well.**

Each and every work mentioned above results from hours upon hours of research culminating in incredibly valuable scholarship to support the claims. These books are very meticulously thought out. Most of the authors have sincere intentions toward helping promote good health as well as procuring some financial reward. And rightfully so, because the provision of this much needed knowledge will not be researched out by the readers; they have nowhere near time nor the gumption, mostly the gumption. Yet, the urgency for this valuable information and direction is unquestionable, regardless if the "readers-in-need" realize the immediate necessity for adopting a reasonably healthy design for eating. Eventually, we are talking about a quality life, because "Father Time" does indeed close the gap between youth and old age. The older you become, the more imperative your food choices measure up to quality nutrients, while avoiding being of the inflammatory nature.

Unfortunately, youth is wasted on the young, who feel bullet-proof and have no fear of eating irresponsibly. By the time wisdom, knowledge, and reason catch up to them, obesity or old age (maybe both) has arrived with all its ailments. The reality is: for some it's too late; their diseases, ailments, or obesity cannot be reversed. That evolution is fatal. This book is not for the under 45 years of age group; those will only question the validity of this dissertation since they have no visible ailments. These are hardcore skeptics with no access to real knowledge.

If you read the "Foreword," you know I am a personal fitness trainer and rehabilitative exercise specialist. Working "for hire" at a community fitness center combined with a senior citizen recreation-activity facility for 15 years has opened my eyes beyond what I previously believed. I have had the misfortune of knowing healthy men and women (on the surface) at ages 45-50 and watching them hit the bottom at 60-65. They have gone from working out in the fitness center to playing dominos in the senior center, using a walker or scooter to get there. Six of my beloved clients have died of disease during this time. All the schemes to change your body from obese to skinny cannot prevent the slide. There are as many crippled lean people as there are disabled overweight people. Therefore, let me please emphasize, body composition evolving from unfavorable to favorable is no indication of a healthy body and brain. Dr. Russell Blaylock (renowned Neurosurgeon) will explain inflammation and its unseen devastation in the following chapter. Hopefully it will alarm you.

It's easy to accept weightlifting as 30% of the process for good health and a judicious diet as 70%. Almost everyone can agree with that, but they cannot find the time to work out, and are too stressed out to eat properly. We live in a technological world that is running at breakneck speed with increasing demands on our body and mind. Our answer to the imposing question about finding time to work out and eat nutritiously is: 'As soon as I find time,' or 'If I can just get a few of these things done.' It never happens – there is no perfect time to begin the groundwork to prevent the inevitable mudslide that washes your body and mind to oblivion.

Like the book's narration, this introduction is short and to-the-point. The goal here amounts to simplifying intelligent food choices in an effort to live a healthy life and stave off disease. With **INFLAMMATION** now the inarguable "father of all disease," it will be necessary to examine the scientific explanations. Alarmingly, an overwhelming number of nutritious whole foods are the culprit and architect of this "deadly" condition. In addition, the three most dangerous processed food additives, **trans fatty acids (TFAs), high fructose corn syrup (HFCS), and MSG (monosodium glutamate)** also spearhead the expeditious development of inflammation. These (known as excitotoxins) too will be discussed, including the science, foods they occupy, and "secret" names manufacturers use on labels.

Just how dangerous is inflammation? Unanimous hard scientific data unequivocally blames this guy for:

- Osteoarthritis
- Rheumatoid arthritis
- Eczema or psoriasis
- Asthma
- Allergies
- Heart disease
- High blood pressure
- High cholesterol
- Alzheimer's disease
- Parkinson's disease
- Diabetes
- Cancer
- Joint pain or stiffness

As a sidelight, for those interested in blood sugar effects of the various carbohydrates, a short section will explain the term "glycemic load," which has replaced the outdated "glycemic index." This is very important for those who judiciously fear diabetes.

There are neither daily meal plans nor recipes offered, but the foods listed do come with portion sizes. There is no need for counting calories. Eating was not meant to be a complex task, where preparation requires a well-equipped laboratory with food weight scales and calculators. Planning necessary to shop for grub should not be a monumental challenge. The victuals outlined in this work are divided into two groups; inflammatory causing (pro-inflammatory) and anti-inflammatory promoting. Every food will have what researchers refer to as an IF Rating (Inflammatory Rating) to go along with a glycemic load indication (GL). The inflammatory food will be designated with a minus sign in front of its number. The anti-inflammatory food will be designated by a positive number; no plus sign.

To graze strictly from the whole food anti-inflammatory group, ensures avoiding inflammation as well as escaping HFCS, TFAs, MSG, counting calories, worrying about carbohydrates, and concerning one's self with portion sizes. However, there are popular nutritious whole foods that are inflammatory, and the task of the reader is to simply juggle the food choices in such a way as to stay on the positive side - anti-inflammatory. In other words, at the end of the day, week, or month, your IF Rating should average out on the plus side. For example, if on a given day you consume two foods that together total -30 and follow with two foods whose rating together adds up to a 50, then your total for the day was a successful 20. How hard could that be? A section on sample meals with similar food choices is presented; one pro-inflammatory and the other anti-inflammatory by changing one item. Another small section presents the worst choices, and still one more offers the **Great Equalizers**; food items so high on the anti-inflammatory scale, they can more than offset a would-be pro-inflammation meal. And by the way, for those concerned about body image, you too will be happy. Those not concerned with body image will just have to accept not being obese.

The real problem amongst the pro-inflammatory lists lies within the processed foods. Here is where the deadliest of the silent assassins reside, lurking in the shadows.

Hope you find the content of this text informative and easy to read and understand.

Stay positive, my friend.

> Honesty is the first chapter in
> the book of Wisdom.
>
> -Thomas Jefferson

BAYLOR SPORTS MEDICINE INSTITUTE

Recognizes

Robin Dobbins

For successfully demonstrating nationally accepted requirements through a comprehensive examination of theoretical knowledge and practical applications for personal training of the general, apparently healthy population, the above named is hereby recognized as a

Certified Personal Fitness Trainer

BSMI-CPFT

Valid Through
07/31/2002

Director of Certification Services

Director of PFT Education Programs

Director of BSMI Certification

BAYLOR SPORTS
MEDICINE INSTITUTE

BAYLOR SPORTS MEDICINE INSTITUTE

Recognizes

Robin Dobbins

For successfully demonstrating nationally accepted requirements through a comprehensive examination of theoretical knowledge and practical applications of advanced understanding and enhanced skills in rehabilitative exercise continuums for the specialized needs of a general, apparently healthy population having experienced an acute or chronic injury, the above named is hereby recognized as a

Rehabilitative Exercise Specialist-Certified
BSMI-RES-C

Valid Through

10/31/03

William M. Brigham, MD
Director of Certification

Sheila S. Hurst
Director of Certification Services

D. Wayne D.
Director of PRT Education Programs

■ BAYLOR SPORTS
■ MEDICINE INSTITUTE

What is inflammation?

Inflammation is the first response of your immune system to infection or irritation (also injury). All of us are familiar with the classic signs of this condition (swelling, redness and pain). Blood and fluid rush to the injured site transporting healing nutrients.

This defense mechanism comes to the rescue when your body's surveillance system detects a foreign body, such as bacterium or virus (infection), invading its territory. Redness and swelling around an infected region is caused by millions of white blood cells speeding toward a site with the purpose of overpowering an intruder. The presence of fever indicates a sort of whole-body inflammation predicated to overcoming the menace. By raising the temperature of the body significantly, the bug will succumb to heatstroke.

Through a sprained ankle (irritation and injury), you have probably witnessed another impressive display of the body's response. An ankle can swell to the size of a melon within minutes, functioning to act as a splint for protective immobilization. As any orthopedist will tell you, doctors don't heal sprained ankles; they just supervise while nature and time do their jobs. Pain is nothing more than a signal to stop what you're doing, thereby avoiding further damage.

These examples of inflammation have a useful purpose, and the swelling gradually subsides and vanishes. No harm; job done.

Undesirable Inflammation
Not in Your Control

Obviously, you don't want to diminish the body's protective and healing powers. But it's a must to eliminate excessive, chronic, and inappropriate inflammation. All kinds of arthritis, for example, are characterized by painful swelling and stiffness in joints. Allergies are another sort of non-productive inflammatory responses in which the immune system tries to attack otherwise harmless substances like pollen or animal dander. These kinds of inflammation serve no useful purpose and can make your life miserable. Over time, excessive inflammation (whatever the cause) increases your risk of several life-threatening diseases, **but at least you are aware of such attacks from inflammation.**

Undesirable Inflammation
In Your Control (Food Consumption)

Recent research has shown eating the wrong foods does cause chronic inflammation within our bodies (at the cellular level). This chronic inflammation is not so obvious. It is the dreaded, more dangerous form – a silent, invisible assassin that destroys every facet of your body (yes, especially the brain) for years without revealing the slightest symptom. Eventually, though, the damage will expose itself in the form of heart disease, Alzheimer's disease, or cancer, to name a few.

Our cells produce a variety of pro and anti-inflammatory chemicals called prostaglandins, using nutrients from the food we eat as the raw material. These prostaglandins are released into our tissues, responding to the immune system's signals, promoting inflammation where there is danger and quelling inflammation, when the danger has passed.

In the April 2010 issue of the **Blaylock Wellness Report**, the prominent neurosurgeon Dr. Russell Blaylock writes:

"There is growing evidence that chronic, smoldering inflammation is a major cause of frailty in the elderly. Remember – where there is inflammation there is massive generation of free radicals and lipid peroxidation products (caustic fats) that are flooding the body – every organ and tissue. They always go together.

These nasty particles and caustic fats not only destroy parts of cells, they also destroy the glue that holds us together – that is, our ligaments, bones, joints, and connective tissue of our skin (causing wrinkles).

Over time, our tissues and organs become so weakened that we begin to break apart like wet sand on a beach. This process doesn't happen overnight; it happens over decades."

This is a rather ugly, gruesome depiction of the reality surrounding this "skipped over" subject matter involving the foods we eat. Dr. Blaylock will be heard from again in this book.

A key concept in this oversimplified portrayal is our bodies produce prostaglandins by using compounds from the foods we eat. Specifically, it is the fatty acids in our foods which our bodies use to make prostaglandins. Certain types of fatty acids (primarily those from the Omega 6 family) are converted into pro-inflammatory prostaglandins, while other types (primarily from the Omega 3 family) are used to make anti-inflammatory prostaglandins. Also, but not minimally, inflammation does develop through diets dominated by processed/packaged foods filled with the three most lethal food additives mentioned in the Introduction: monosodium glutamate, high fructose corn syrup, and trans fatty acids. Mercifully, nature has provided the antidote; foods that are just as effective at reversing inflammation.

Conditions Characterized by Excessive Inflammation Regardless of the Cause

- Heart Disease
- Alzheimer's disease
- Cancer
- Obesity
- Diabetes
- Autoimmune Diseases
- Asthma
- Allergies

- Arthritis
- Prostate Disease

The "IF" (Inflammatory) System to the Rescue

The "IF" Rating system was developed in an effort to make it easier for a non-specialist to understand the inflammatory or anti-inflammatory effects facilitated by a wide variety of foods. Each is given an "IF" rating number, representing the net inflammatory or anti-inflammatory impact of that food.

The "good guys" are foods represented by a positive number, and the "bad guys" have a negative designation. IF ratings between 1 and 100 possess mildly anti-inflammatory properties. Numbers between 101 and 500 are moderately anti-inflammatory, and those over 500 are strongly anti-inflammatory. On the other end of the scale, numbers ranging between -1 and -100 are mildly inflammatory. Foods ranging between -101 and -500 prove to be moderately inflammatory, and ones showing -500 and above are considered strongly inflammatory. It makes sense these two rosters are made available in this book and should be the backbone to simplify your making good decisions concerning eating healthy foods, while avoiding horrific disease causing inflammatory ones. Poor decisions will catch up to you; make no mistake. Should you have doubts or be a mighty skeptic, be more observant when venturing out to the grocery store or settling in at your favorite restaurant. Go to a fitness center and take inventory of whose participating in water aerobics. Crippling obesity dominates the scene, but amazingly, those few who look fit and trim may be just as disabled. So feast your eyes upon those aforementioned, because they are mirroring what you will look like some day should inflammation causing foods heavily dot your meals and snacks. Roll the dice with boisterous flare, but you will be the loser.

How the IF Rating is Calculated

The IF Rating integrates more than twenty (20) different pro-inflammatory and anti-inflammatory factors. The amounts of individual nutrients are considered, as well as the ratios between various nutrients. The formula also incorporates the glycemic load, which describes the impact a food has on blood sugar; whether it causes blood sugar to rise sharply or slowly. It also takes into consideration processed/packaged foods (especially) containing a relatively new concept: "**excitotoxins;**" monosodium glutamate, high fructose corn syrup, and trans fats being the main culprits.

Where does all of this information come from? The U.S. Department of Agriculture. The USDA has conducted extensive nutritional analyses on thousands of raw, processed, and commercially prepared foods. These measurements make up the National Nutritional Database for Standard Reference and are used as the basis of virtually all nutritional databases in our country. The most recent update for the database (SR17) was published in 2004 and provides considerable details used in calculations of those IF Ratings.

Determining Your Level of Systemic Inflammation

C-reactive protein (CRP) is a compound in the blood signaling the presence of nonspecific systemic inflammation. Elevated levels of CRP are a serious warning inflammation is gathering significantly somewhere in the body. Fortunately, there are medical tests that can measure the presence of inflammation long before a serious disease has developed. This can be done with a rather affordable, reliable blood test, which has become the most widely used measure of systemic inflammation.

Fibrinogen, a compound that indicates the propensity of blood to form clots, is sometimes used as a secondary indication inflammation is present, especially in heart patients. As with CRP, higher levels of fibrinogen suggest increased inflammation. And most recently, researchers have discovered elevated white blood cell counts indicate an increased risk of inflammation related disease, particularly in women. Different test combinations can provide a physician with a nuanced picture of the patient's inflammatory processes. In general, however, a simple CRP test is entirely sufficient to screen for and track the presence of systemic inflammation. Many physicians will include a CRP test in your annual blood workup if you ask. In fact, it is recommended those over forty (40) have this done, especially if you have a family history of the diseases referred to in these narrations.

Understanding Your Test Results

The CRP test is not a test for any particular disease or condition. It will not state whether you have heart disease, cancer, or Alzheimer's disease. This test will simply indicate whether you have an excessive level of systemic inflammation.

CRP is usually measured in milligrams per liter (mg/L). Ideally you want your CRP levels to be in the "no risk" to "slightly risky" range (.55-1.14) for men and "no risk" (<1.5) for women. As you can see, in the table provided, even slight elevations of CRP have been tied to an increased risk of heart attack, stroke, and other diseases.

Important Note: Any infection or injury will cause a temporary rise in your CRP levels as the body's immune system responds to the crisis. If you experience an acute infection or injury, wait two weeks before scheduling a CRP test to ensure an accurate result.

CRP Levels and Disease Risks

Men

CPR	**Risk of Future Heart Attack**
0.55 mg/L or less	No increased risk; ideal
0.56-1.14 mg/L	Slightly more likely
1.15-2.10 mg/L	2 ½ times as likely
2.11 mg/L and higher	3 times as likely

Women

CRP	**Risk of Future Heart Attack or Stroke**
Less than 1.50 mg/L	No increased risk; Ideal
1.50-3.79 mg/L	2 ½ times as likely
3.80-7.30 mg/L	3 ½ times as likely
7.31 mg/L and higher	5 ½ times as likely

Monosodium Glutamate (MSG)

Monosodium glutamate is a naturally occurring salt form of glutamate, which makes it highly absorbable. But it is the glutamate in MSG that causes toxicity. All forms of glutamate, natural or artificial, are equally harmful if glutamate (glutamic acid) is isolated.

The difference is natural glutamate found in whole foods rarely appears alone. It is always combined with other substances to create a complex protein. For natural glutamate to be released, it must experience digestion. This releases the glutamate slowly, allowing the body time to deal with it safely.

Cooking high-glutamate foods, such as red meats, tomatoes, and mushrooms, allows the glutamate to be released and even concentrated - as in meat juices (broth and stocks) and vegetable extracts (hydrolyzed proteins and soy protein isolates and extracts). These forms of glutamate can be just as toxic as MSG.

In the words of Dr. Russell Blaylock, a nationally recognized, board-certified neurosurgeon, health practitioner, author, and lecturer; "When I first wrote my book, 'Excitotoxins: The Taste That Kills,' scientists were just beginning to learn how glutamate damaged the nervous system and the brain. Since then, we have learned an enormous amount about the function of glutamate in the brain and how it can cause damage - sometimes permanent when present in excess amounts."

In 1969, neuroscientist Dr. John Olney of the Washington University School of Medicine first discovered the manner in which excess glutamate destroys brains cells. He called this process **excitotoxicity**. Dr. Olney called the process by this name because when he added small amounts of monosodium glutamate to brain cells in a culture, the cells began to shrivel up and die after about an hour. He noted that just before this happened, the neurons were firing very rapidly, suggesting they were burning up themselves. Hence the name combining the root words excito (excite) and toxicity (poison).

Glutamate receptors (glutamate) are now being shown to play a major role in a growing list of neurological and psychiatric disorders, including:

- Alzheimer's
- Parkinson's
- ALS, Huntington's
- Depression
- Anxiety
- Schizophrenia
- Obsessive - Compulsive Disorder

- Autism
- ADHD
- Chronic Pain
- Addiction
- Strokes
- Brain Injury

There is also a host of other health issues and dangers prevalent with MSG. This flavor enhancer is linked to:

- Fibromyalgia
- Obesity
- Fatty liver
- High insulin and blood sugar
- High cholesterol
- Liver toxicity
- Metabolic syndrome
- High blood pressure
- Disturbance to the gut-brain connection
- Neurological and brain damage

Hidden Names for MSG and Free Glutamic Acid

- Glutamic Acid
- Glutamate
- Monosodium Glutamate
- Monopotassium Glutamate
- Calcium Glutamate
- Monoammonium Glutamate
- Magnesium Glutamate
- Natrium Glutamate
- Yeast Extract
- Anything hydrolyzed
- Any hydrolyzed protein
- Calcium Caseinate
- Sodium Caseinate
- Yeast Food
- Yeast Nutrient
- Autolyzed Yeast
- Gelatin
- Textured Protein
- Soy Protein
- Soy Protein Concentrate
- Soy Protein Isolate
- Whey Protein
- Whey Protein Concentrate
- Whey Protein Isolate
- Anything protein
- Vetsin
- Ajinomoto

Names of Ingredients That Often Contain Manufactured Free Glutamic Acid

- Carrageenan
- Bouillon and broth
- Stock
- Any flavors or flavoring
- Maltodextrin
- Citric acid, Citrate
- Anything ultra-pasteurized
- Barley malt
- Pectin
- Protease
- Anything enzyme modified
- Anything containing enzymes
- Malt extract
- Soy sauce
- Soy sauce extract
- Anything protein fortified
- Anything fermented
- Seasonings

A number of natural substances found in plant based diets have been shown to be very **protective** against excitotoxicity. These include:

- Magnesium
- Selenium

- Vitamin B6
- Mixed tocopherols and tocotrienols
- B vitamins
- Methylcobalamin
- Folate
- Flavanoids
- Silymarin
- Baicalein
- Grape seed extract
- DHA
- Vitamin D3
- Hawthorn extract

The Science

Glutamate has been discovered to be the most abundant transmitter in the brain, accounting for more than 90% of the communication in the brain's cortex and more than 50% of all the grey matter's communication. Glutamate transmissions exceed those of all the other transmitters, such as acetylcholine, serotonin, dopamine, and norepinephrine combined. We're talking here about the glutamate inside the cell walls.

In the words of Dr. Blaylock, "Glutamate damages the brain cells only it if is outside the cell where the receptors are located. This glutamate comes from our food, especially the manufactured MSG. God equipped our brains with a number of protective mechanisms that keep glutamate mostly within brain cells. The ratio of inside to outside the brain cell is 1,000 to 1."

A number of other mechanisms also help protect the brain, most of which require a lot of energy. Brain disorders such as stroke, trauma, neurodegenerative diseases (Alzheimer's, Parkinson's), and heavy metal poisoning result in a loss of brain energy. People with these disorders risk damage to the brain from even small exposures to dietary excitotoxins.

As we age, our brain energy decreases, and protective systems begin to falter. The brain then becomes progressively more inflamed. Together, these factors make us extra sensitive to dietary excitotoxins, and our brains begin to leak glutamate from storage sites, primarily the glia, which are the brain's immune cells. This is why the incidence of Alzheimer's goes from 3%, at age 65, to 50% at age 80.

Exposure to high levels of glutamic acid in the diet may also explain the explosion of obesity among the young and even among older people. MSG additives via processed foods were introduced to the public on a grand scale in 1948. Now they are out of control, as virtually every major food manufacturer uses some other form of the excitotoxic additive, especially trans fats and high fructose corn syrup. When excitotoxic food additives are ingested, they take a journey from the gastrointestinal tract to the liver via the portal vein. This makes the liver very vulnerable to damage, because it is exposed to the highest concentration of glutamate. Studies have shown that dietary MSG significantly raises inflammation, and causes a massive production of free radicals and lipid peroxidation in the liver that can persist for a very long time. This increases the damage from other toxins.

Glutamate is also a cancer fertilizer and can alter the function of every cell in the body. Recent studies have shown glutamate is found in every tissue and organ in the body, including:

- Skin and bones
- GI tract
- Pancreas
- Liver
- Kidney
- Reproductive organs (testes and ovaries)
- Prostate
- Immune cells

When folks are sensitive to MSG, they are actually reacting to **free** glutamic acid in the blood. Remember, MSG is made when the **free** glutamic acid binds with a sodium molecule. Whenever protein is broken down in the body, glutamic acid is **freed** from a protein in which it naturally occurs. Consequently, you have the potential of free glutamic acid building up in the blood and a possible toxic MSG reaction.

While this happens naturally, when ingesting protein-rich whole foods like grains, meats, dairy, and even vegetables, the glutamic acid is released in concert with many other amino acids, rather than in high concentrations on its own. As a result, unadulterated whole-food-based proteins do not cause a toxic MSG reaction in the body.

On the other hand, many processed foods, including organic health foods, contain processed proteins that harbor free glutamic acids (toxins).

Remember, glutamic acid found in unadulterated "whole food" protein does not cause adverse reactions. To cause adverse reactions, the glutamic acid must have been processed/manufactured or come from protein that has been fermented.

The Beginning

MSG, or monosodium glutamate, got its reputation as a flavor enhancer extracted from seaweeds in China. The year 1908 saw the process perfected in Japan by Professor Kikunae Ikeda and became commercially available. Concentrated free glutamic acid or MSG act as nerve stimulants and will change how the taste buds embrace the food. A yucky or even a really foul flavored food will taste fantastic when high levels of glutamic acid are introduced.

In the 1960's, the phrase "Chinese Restaurant Syndrome" was coined by the New England Journal of Medicine. Twenty minutes after eating Chinese food, some people sensitive to MSG would experience tingling, numbness, brain fog, chest pressure, and pain.

By the 1970's, researchers found that pharmaceutical MSG would kill brain cells in a laboratory. Shortly thereafter, they realized commercially available MSG had the same effect.

Do you need any more convincing to by-pass the center aisles when touring the grocery store? Jack LaLane, one of the pioneers of health and fitness, once said, "If it's packaged, I don't eat it."

High Fructose Corn Syrup

The corn industry is desperately attempting to convince the public (as well as the FDA) high fructose corn syrup (HFCS) is a "natural" product and no more harmful for human consumption than cane sugar. "Corn people" argue their product is not the culprit it is made out to be. It has been acknowledged by all contending parties too much of either is bad. However, Dr. Bruce Ames, a renowned professor of Biochemistry and Molecular Biology Emeritus at the University of California, Berkley, and a senior scientist at Children's Hospital Oakland Research Institute has **shared** shocking new evidence from his research center how HFCS can trigger body-wide inflammation and obesity.

It is necessary to understand some basic biochemistry. Regular cane sugar (sucrose) is made of two-sugar molecules bound tightly together - glucose and fructose in equal amounts. The enzymes in your digestive tract must break down the sucrose into glucose and fructose, which are then absorbed into the body.

HFCS also consists of glucose and fructose. However, it is not in a 50/50 ratio, but a 55/45 fructose to glucose ratio in an **unbound form**. Fructose is sweeter than glucose. Since there is **no chemical bond** between them, digestion is not required, allowing both to more rapidly be absorbed into your blood stream. Fructose goes straight to the liver and triggers lipogenesis, the production of fats (triglycerides) and cholesterol. **This is why high fructose corn syrup is the major cause of liver damage in this country.** "Fatty Liver" affects over 70 million people. The rapidly absorbed glucose triggers big spikes in insulin - our body's major fat storage hormone. Both of these features of HFCS lead to increased metabolic disturbances that drive increase appetites, weight gain, diabetes, heart disease, cancer, accelerated aging, dementia, and more.

Also, high doses of free fructose (from HFCS) have been proven to literally punch holes in the intestinal lining, allowing **nasty** by-products of toxic gut bacteria and partially digested food proteins to enter your blood stream and ignite the inflammation that we know is at the root of all disease. **Naturally occurring fructose in fruit is part of a complex of nutrients and fiber that does not exhibit the same biological effects as the free high fructose doses found in "corn sugar."**

Production

Corn syrups, including HFCS, are made from corn starch. Commercial production of corn syrup began in 1864. During the late 1950's, scientists at Clinton Corn Processing Company in Iowa tried to transform glucose from corn starch into fructose, but the process was not scalable. In 1965 Yoshiyuki Tasasaki at the Japanese National Institute of Advanced Industrial Science and Technology (AIST) developed a heat-stable xylose isomerase enzyme from yeast, and three years later AIST partnered with the Clinton Company to successfully commercialize the process.

In the contemporary process, corn (maize) is milled to produce corn starch, and an "acid-enzyme" process is used causing the corn starch solution to become acidified to begin breaking up the existing carbohydrates. The corn starch is further metabolized to convert the resulting sugars into fructose. The first enzyme added is alpha-amylase which breaks the long chains down into shorter sugar chains - oligosaccharides. Glucoamylase is mixed in and converts them into glucose. The resulting solution is filtered to remove protein, using activated carbon, and then demineralized, using ion-exchange resins. The purified solution is then run over immobilized xylose isomerase, which turns the sugars to 50-52% glucose with some unconverted oligosaccharides, and 42% fructose (HFCS 42), and again demineralized and again purified using activated carbon. Some is processed into HFCS 90 by liquid chromatology, then mixed with HFCS 42 to form HFCS 55. The enzymes used in the process are made by microbial fermentation.

If one fully follows this process, he or she is far ahead of my understanding. For myself, this was an exercise in futility; simply one to validate this short essay on a food researchers agree is highly toxic (especially with mercury).

Historical Background

Prior to the development of the worldwide sugar industry, dietary fructose was limited to only a few items. Milk, meats, and most vegetables, the staples of many early diets, have no fructose, and only 5-10% fructose by weight is found in fruits such as grapes, apples, blueberries. From 1970 to 2000 there was a 25% increase in added sugars in the U.S. After being classified as "generally recognized as safe," (GRAS) by the U.S. Food & Drug Administration in1976, HFCS began to replace sucrose (cane sugar) as the main sweetener in soft drinks in the U.S. by 1984. At the same time, obesity escalated.

HFCS is used worldwide as a sweetener due to being easier to handle than granulated sugar and less expensive due to the price of the raw material, corn, being subsidized by the government.

Trans Fatty Acids (TFAs)

According to a distressing report (July 2002) by the Institute of Medicine at the National Academy of Sciences, our government's adviser to health policy, Americans are ingesting foods with an ingredient which has zero acceptable levels of consumption - trans fatty acids (TFAs). This declaration resulted in the FDA handing down labeling requirements forcing manufacturers of processed foods to reveal the presence of this venomous additive by 2006.

Trans fatty acids are manufactured through a process called **hydrogenation**. Soy beans, safflower seeds, grapeseed (Canola), cottonseeds, corn, and sunflower seeds are crushed, producing pure vegetable oils. At this point, these oils are good for you as fatty acids. Now begins the poisonous process, honing the oils with chemical solvents to deodorize and bleach. A metal catalyst (ordinarily nickel) is added to speed up the chemical reaction of this solution. From there, the brew is subjected to extremely high pressure and heat, coupled with injection of hydrogen gas. Presto, you have a molecular reaction that produces a solid product at room temperature; no longer an oil at all, but a thick plastic.

These manufactured unnatural fats absolutely cause dysfunction - a Chinese Fire Drill at the cellular level in your body. The consequences of consistent consumption of TFAs are accumulatively catastrophic.

Cells in our bodies are distinguished by membranes, which are thin semi-permeable coverings enclosing a cell's contents. A membrane's function is to preserve the integrity of the cell by allowing certain substances to enter and chasing away others. These rascals are composed of oils, some protein, and various carbohydrates. The oils are continually renewed and replaced. Therefore, the human body's functions depend upon the oils we consume on a daily basis.

Cells must be flexible and respond instantly to hormones, inflammation, and other changes. The **flexibility** depends upon the kinds of oils allowed to enter the body. This flexibility enhances the presentation of the proper targets for which chemical messengers coordinate paramount bodily functions.

When **partially hydrogenated oils** (TFAs) stumble into our food intake, they too enter the cell membrane. The plastic TFAs also take up cell space preventing good fats from entering. Consequently, crucial membrane flexibility is replaced by stiffness, causing loss of ability to signal and respond effectively to life's requirements. Eventually, the human body will begin to break down. Inflammation of the cells begins to spread, causing innumerable metabolic nightmares.

What are these nightmares? How about embracing insulin resistance (Type II Diabetes), obesity, heart disease, autoimmune disease, cancer, asthma, bone degeneration, reproductive problems, cholesterol problems (lowering the "good" and increasing the "bad), and depression? Sound good? If so, keep eating the following:

All Packaged or Processed Foods
Examples:

Breakfast Cereals	Quaker Oats Chewy Granola Bars
Saltine Crackers	Special K's entire line of health/ weight loss food
Girl Scout Cookies	Pop Corn (Microwavable)
Animal Crackers	Fig Newtons (except fat-free version)
Ritz Crackers	Fortune Cookies

Frozen Pies, Pot Pies, Pie Crust   Frozen Pizza, Tacos
Many hamburger and hot dog   Cheesecake, Cornbread, Brownies
buns
Any restaurant food cooked

The good news is TFAs will be eliminated from your cells when you no longer eat foods comprising such. Given the opportunity, healthy fatty acids will eventually replace those horrible TFAs and more efficient cell function will be reinstated. The bad news is structural damage already done cannot be reversed.

It is true that much information in the field of health changes so often, one may hope someday there is some good in TFAs; that they're really not as bad as first thought. Unfortunately, the possibility here does not exist - ever. The substance is plastic.

It must also be noted that the FDA food label ruling on TFAs left the food manufacturers a slight "loop hole;" as long as the food has less than .50 grams of trans fat per serving, the label is allowed to read "0". That means .49 is legal per serving. This adds up quickly considering few people actually consume just one serving of any food.

Why do restaurants, especially fast food establishments, prefer to cook with trans fat? They're cheap, can be used and continually reused, besides making fried foods crispier. The cost effective list is simply infinite.

Historical Background

The great Industrial Revolution of the late nineteenth century caused an enormous migration of rural people around the world to the urban manufacturing centers. This swell created unpredictable circumstances, especially for those seeking their fortune while leaving "the farm." Severe food shortages, housing scarcity, poor sanitation and health dominated the landscape along with crime.

New York City was a crowded slum rampant with disease, and the poor, uneducated, and hungry were poised for terrifying municipal unrest and gang wars. Paris saw people living on the verge of starvation. One slum outside Paris was referred to as the Siberia of Paris. Artisans and assembly line workers were frequently in distress with twelve hour days of hard labor, poor living conditions, and poor diet. Similar conditions existed in England and the rest of Europe.

Food shortages and the lack of animal fat for cooking were the monumental concerns. The French government led the way with huge sums of money toward grants for urging its scientists to solve the problems of food spoilage and the lack of fat with which to cook or bake. Food substitutes and preservation were the priorities.

One food the working class could not afford was animal fat - beef, butter, poultry fat, and lard from pigs. This scarcity meant the loss of an essential cooking and baking ingredient.

Napoleon III offered huge financial gifts to French scientists, encouraging the climate of investigation. A French chemist named Hippolyte Mege-Marries invented a product made completely from animal parts. Using an acid called margaric as part of the process, he named the miracle product margarine.

However, this margarine did not resemble butter nor lard which it was designed to replace. Unattractive and brownish in color, it was prone to becoming rancid. It also had the unfortunate fragrance of rendered meat parts. Though somewhat more affordable, it was still too expensive to produce. A new focus became crucial - how to replace this with something that would not spoil and yet less expensive to render.

In 1897, two French chemists, Jean Sabatier and Jean-Baptiste Sendrens, discovered there was more hydrogen in solid animal fats than vegetable oils. They wondered what would happen if hydrogen was added to vegetable oil. Could it make margarine?

Wilhelm Norman, a German scientist, heard about Sabatier's theory (an article) in 1901. He was able to transform liquid oleic acid (later known as oleo margarine) into solid stearic acid by the use of hydrogen and dispersed nickel. This was the precursor of saturated fat hardening. On February 27, 1901, he finalized the process and on August 14, 1902, secured a patent. From 1901 to 1909 he was head of the laboratory at Leprince & Siveke, where he conducted investigations of the properties of fats and oils.

TFAs were a miracle solution for food preservation and inexpensive cooking and baking oils for the poor. These oils needed no refrigeration, and foods processed with them could last years on the shelf. Long shelf life solved the problem of food shortages.

The Truth About TFAs; Why It Took So Long

In 1913, Proctor & Gamble, makers of Ivory soap, began to market Crisco. It was the first edible food product other than margarine manufactured with hydrogenated oils. It leaped in popularity during WWI and WWII due to animal fat and meat rationing. By the 1950s, the American Heart Association announced the United States was in the midst of a coronary heart disease epidemic. Once the cause of such was discovered, Crisco and other hydrogenated cooking oils were a Godsend.

When in 1956, President Eisenhower initiated the interstate highway system legislation, packaged foods could be transported across the nation and overseas without fear of spoilage.

But a biochemist named Mary Enig and a few concerned physicians in the late 1970s began to question whether there were adverse effects from manufactured trans fatty acids. Was the human body liking them?

Of course not, but the cover-up lasted over 20 years due to one and only one major reason: money. No one was falling down in the street and dying. The effects could not be seen on the surface. The food industry had too much money invested in hydrogenated oils for food preservation and preparation. The oils were cheap and profits higher. They had powerful lobbyists covering Congressional committees like an umbrella. It took record heart disease victims and other deadly health problems surfacing to go along with dedicated researchers persevering to bring the cause of this fatal ingredient in our food supply to light.

Sample Meal Plans Comparisons

BREAKFAST:

Bad Choice   **IF Rating**

Eggs (Whole) 4 Oz   -170

Bacon (Pan Fried) 3 Oz   -36

Blueberry Muffin (1 Muffin)   -75

                                                -281

Good Choice

Eggs, Whole (4 Oz)   -170

Pan Fried Bacon (3 Oz)   -36

Hot Chili Peppers (1/2 Cup)   1,024

Red Grapefruit (1/2 Fruit)   10

                                                828

Bad Choice

Eggs (Whole) 4 Oz   -170

Ham Spiral Cut Roasted (3 Oz)   -32

English Muffin Mixed Grain (1 Muffin)   -39

                                                -241

Good Choice	**IF Rating**
Scrambled Egg Substitutes	20
Cayenne Pepper (1/2 Tsp)	254
Polish Sausage (Pork)	19
Red Grapefruit (1/2 Fruit)	10
	303

Bad Choice	
Eggs Whites (6 Oz)	-6
Turkey Bacon (3 Oz)	-206
French Toast w/o Syrup	-30
	-242

Good Choice	
Omelette	
Egg Whites (6 Oz)	-6
Jalapeno Raw (1/2 Cup)	825
Ham Slice Extra Lean	2
Fat Free Mozzarella	20
	841

LUNCH OR DINNER:

Bad Choice	IF Rating
Roasted Chicken Breast	-25
Kidney Beans (Canned)	-66
Beets (Canned)	-6
	-97

Good Choice	IF Rating
Roasted Chicken Breast	-25
Sweet Potato Baked	189
Asparagus Cooked	38
	202

Bad Choice	
Chicken Wings Roasted	-56
Brown Rice	-143
Turnip Greens	-1
	-200

Good Choice	
Chicken Wings Roasted	-56
Broccoli Cooked	60
Butternut Squash Baked	91
	95

Bad Choice	
Deer Loin Roasted	-99
Corn on the Cobb	-111
Black-eyed Peas (Canned w/Pork)	-86
	-296

Good Choice	IF Rating
Deer Loin Roasted	-99
Spinach Cooked	224
Carrots Cooked	130
	255

Bad Choice	
Pork Top Loin Broiled	-18
Baked Potato w/Skin (White)	-47
Pinto Beans (Canned)	-87
	-152

Good Choice	
Pork Top Sirloin Broiled	-18
Mustard Greens Cooked	172
Okra Cooked	10
	164

The Worst Choices

Starchy Vegetables	IF Rating
Pumpkin (Canned)	-68
Corn on the Cobb	-111
Cooked	-76
Creamed Canned	-56
Potato-Mashed	-69
Hash Brown	-93

Non-Starchy Vegetables
NONE

Fruits	
Blueberries Dried/Sweetened	-120
Heavy Syrup	-70
Syrup Drained	-65
Blackberries Heavy Syrup	-65
Boysenberries Heavy Syrup	-65
Peaches Dried	-76
Banana Chips Dried	-132
Pineapple Frozen Sweet	-64
Plums Heavy Syrup	-70

	IF Rating
Raisins	-135
Seedless	-135
Cherries Maraschino	-122
Frozen Sweet	-76
Tart Dried/Sweet	-143
Sweet Heavy Syrup	-64
Sour Heavy Syrup	-71
Sour Light Syrup	-63
Pears Dried	-114
Raspberries Frozen Sweet	-64
Heavy Syrup	-65
Prunes Dried	-91
Stewed	-82
Stewed w/Sugar	-114
Cranberries Dried/Sweetened	-98
Papaya Heavy Syrup/Drained	-215

White Rice

	IF Rating
Long Grain Cooked	-153
Instant Cooked	-131
Medium Grain Cooked	-184
Short Grain Cooked	-188

Brown Rice

	IF Rating
Long Grain Cooked	-143
Medium Grain Cooked	-162

Noodles

	IF Rating
Chow Mein	-91
Egg Cooked	-102

Rice Cooked   -150

Spaghetti

White Cooked	-124
Whole Wheat Cooked	-82
Spinach Cooked	-120

Oils

Coconut	-115
Cotton Seed	-94
Palm Kernel	-99
Poppy Seed	-78
Safflower High Linoleic	-91
Sunflower Linoleic	-77
Grapeseed	-87

Nuts

Sunflower Seeds Oil-Roasted	-63
Chestnuts Roasted	-70

Flour (All Averages -180)

Best Bets

Peanut Defatted	-1
Whole Wheat	-89
Oat	-103
Buckwheat	-100
Sesame Seed	-68
Soy Full Fat	-23
Low Fat	-7

Sugar (However GL is outrageous @ 150)	IF Rating
Brown	-77
Granulated	-63

Yogurt (No Good Choices)
Check back of book under (Bad Guys) IF Ratings

Granola (Surprisingly, No Good Choices)
Check back of book under (Bad Guys) IF Ratings

Milk
See back of book under (Bad Guys) IF Ratings

Bread
Sticks Plain	-80
Crumbs	-91
Sourdough	-261

Muffins
Blueberry	-75

Rolls & Biscuits
Cinnamon	-70
Brown & Serve	-61
Biscuits/Mix	-61
Refrigerated Dough	-62
Reduced Fat	-60

Dressings (All are below -50)
Eat what you like

Cookies (No Good Choices)
Check back of book under (Bad Guys) IF Ratings

Ice Cream & Other Desserts (No Good Choices)
Check back of book under (Bad Guys) IF Ratings

Meat

	IF Rating
Beef Heart Simmered	-168
Liver Braised	-233
Pan Fried	-143
Chicken Thigh Batter Fried	-76
Fried	-89
Stewed	-69
Wings Batter Fried	-80
Fried	-93
Stewed	-72
Leg Batter Fried	-73
Fried	-79
Stewed	-67
Chicken Heart Simmered	-502
Giblets Fried	-259
Simmered	-152
Liver Pan Fried	-272
Simmered	-274
Drumstick Batter Fried	-70
Fried	-74
Dark Meat Fried w/o Skin	-97
Roasted w/o Skin	-78
Stewed w/o Skin	-71
Cornish Hens Roasted	-128
Roasted w/o Skin	-128
Pork Ground 72% Lean Cooked	-68
Spareribs Roasted	-64
Bacon Baked	-67
Bacon Microwaved	-91

	IF Rating
Turkey Bacon	-206
Country Style Ham	-78
Deer Loin Roasted	-99
Ground Browned	-60
Elk Roasted	-77
Lamb Ribs Broiled	-77
Turkey Breast Roasted	-104
Giblets Simmered	-136
Ground Cooked	-80
Heart Simmered	-201
Liver Simmered	-184
Leg Roasted	-162
Smoked Turkey	-136
Wing Roasted	-102
Veal Loin Braised	-92
Roasted	-71
Liver Braised	-138
Pan Fried	-160
Rib Braised	-63
Shoulder	-64
Sirloin Braised	-63

Eggs

Chicken Whole	-85
Yolk	-182
Goose	-126
Duck	-147

Beans (Have much nutrition)

Check back of book under (Bad Guys) IF Ratings

The Great Equalizers

The following pages list the outstanding anti-inflammatory foods, illustrating their impact upon a meal dominated by pro-inflammatory ones. There are plenty of pro-inflammatory whole foods we all love to eat which possess numerous important nutrients. With strategically placed **Great Equalizers,** we can enjoy them and still maintain meals rendering an anti-inflammatory rating. Keep in mind, one meal on the pro-inflammatory side of the scale doesn't place you in the stockade. The big picture is what matters; what side of the scale were you at the end of the day, week, or month. If you predominantly eat your meals from the anti-inflammatory side and avoid desserts and processed foods, you'll be in great shape.

Once you venture off into the center aisles of the grocery store, you are on your own. Enter at your own risk. There are very few items in that maze, you can afford to consume without inviting trouble from MSG, HFCS, and trans fats. These three killers are loaded with excitotoxins that cause deadly inflammation and obesity.

Even on the pro-inflammatory side (refer to the back of the book under Bad Guys IF Ratings), there are very few whole foods you should limit due to their inflammatory nature; their rating is low. Note, however, even if all the foods in a meal have extremely low IF ratings, it still renders a pro-inflammatory result. Consistent living on the pro-inflammatory side, no matter how low the rating, leaves the body in a state of inflammation – disease causing.

(The foods on the following pages are all IF Ratings)

FISH (3 Oz)

Striped Bass (Baked)	422
Blue Fish (Baked)	439
Flounder (Baked or Grilled)	204
Anchovy (Canned in Oil)	871
White Fish (Baked)	422
Halibut (Cold Water)	497
Salmon (Wild/Baked)	489
Salmon (Chinook/Baked)	582
Salmon (Canned)	444
Salmon (Sockeye/Baked)	493
Sardines (Atlantic)	435
Sardines (Pacific)	344
Swordfish (Baked)	349
Sea Bass (Baked)	344
Roe (Baked)	1,040
All Oysters	250-300
Mackerel (Atlantic/Baked)	510
Mackerel (Spanish/Baked)	395
Mackerel (Pacific/Baked)	683
Mackerel (Canned)	465
Rainbow Trout Wild (Baked)	308
Tuna Bluefin (Baked)	593
Tuna White (Canned in Water)	344

Note: Farm raised fish are often pro-inflammatory due to their diet being grain instead of algae and small fish.

Vegetables

Spinach	
Canned	241
Cooked	224
Frozen/Cooked	187
Dandelion Greens	
Cooked	131
Raw	150
Turnip Greens/Cooked	238
Mustard Greens/Cooked	172
Sweet Potato/Baked	189
Swiss Chard/Cooked	121
Kale	
Cooked	112
Frozen/Cooked	213
Broccoli/Cooked	60
Collards/Cooked	159
Carrots	
Cooked	130
Raw	98
Onions	
Cooked	240
Frozen/Cooked	301
Raw	292
Sweet Raw	299

Seasonings

Cayenne (1/2 Tsp)	254
Ginger Root (1 Tbsp)	387
Ground Ginger Root (1/2 Tsp)	348
Garlic Raw (1 Tbsp)	215
Garlic Powder (1 Tbsp)	468
Turmeric (1 Tsp)	338

Chili Peppers (1/2 Cup)

Banana Raw	654
Hot Raw	1,024
Hot Sundried	1,366
Hungarian Raw	659
Jalapeno Canned	479
Jalapeno Raw	825
Serrano Raw	1,556
Green Canned	551
Hot Canned	701

Spreads

Almond Butter (1/4 Cup)	100
Peanut Butter w/Omega 3 (2 Tbsp)	91

Bad Meals Saved by the Great Equalizer
Designated by an *

Salmon (Wild/Baked)	489*
Corn on the Cobb	-111
White Baked Potato	-47
Chocolate Ice Cream (1/2 Cup)	-83
	248

Halibut (Cold Water)	497*
Rice Noodles	-150
Blackeyed Peas (Canned)	-86
Cornbread (2 Oz)	-158
	103

Rainbow Trout	308*
Garbanzo (Chick Peas)	-82
Bread Multi-Grain (1 Slice)	-34
Yogurt/Greek Berry (Chobani)	-108
	84

Pan Fried Liver (3 Oz)	-143
Turnip Greens Cooked	238*
Onions Cooked	240*
White Potato Baked	-47
	288

Pan Fried Liver	-143
Onions Cooked	240*
Brown Rice Cooked	-143
Spinach Cooked	224*
	178

Roasted Turkey Leg	-162
White Rice Cooked	-182
White Bread (2 Slices)	-106
Almond Butter	100*
Mustard Greens Cooked	172*
Green Chili Peppers Canned	551*
	373

T-Bone Steak Broiled (6 Oz)	-36
Lima Beans (Cooked)	-45
Carrots Cooked	130*
	49

Blenderize Your Vegetables

According to Dr. Russell Blaylock, a renowned neurosurgeon, health practitioner, author, and lecturer, one should try blenderizing their vegetables. The blender can do a much better job of tearing down the cell walls of the vegetables than your teeth ever dreamed of doing.

In his January 2009 newsletter, Dr. Blaylock says, "Drinking a cup of blenderized vegetable juice is the equivalent to eating eight to ten servings of raw fruits and vegetables. It's estimated that the body absorbs only about 30 percent of nutrients from eating raw, chewed vegetables. Blenderized vegetables are absorbed at a rate of 90 percent."

The following vegetables are important to your blending experience:

- Asparagus
- Carrots
- Spinach
- Broccoli
- Grape Tomatoes
- Cucumbers
- Kale
- Red Cabbage
- Collard Greens
- Cauliflower
- Brussels Sprouts
- Celery
- Parsley

Personally, none of these vegetables thrill my taste buds. However, they have proven to be a powerful force toward preventing a number of cancers. They contain flavonoids that are powerful antioxidants and have anti-inflammatory properties. This is the reason, I even allow them to grace my ever resistant lips. However, you can make a blended recipe bearable.

My recipe is:

- Frozen Strawberries (creates coldness)
- One Banana (cut into small pieces)
- Asparagus
- Broccoli
- Spinach
- Grape Tomatoes
- Carrots

I then pour 20-24 ounces of water down the blender's throat, secure the lid and hit the start button. My Ninja Professional 1000 watt guy then turns everything into liquid; makes 9 cups. I drink 3 cups all at once per day, placing the rest in the fridge, container and all. The three-cup concoction gives me 30 servings of raw fruits and vegetables for each of three days. A nutritionist explained the "stuff" will keep up to 10 days.

Now the pressure is off in terms of getting the proper amounts of fruits and "good" vegetables. I can then concentrate on lean meats and fish while tossing in another vegetable or two at mealtime. The vegetables will also be of the anti-inflammatory variety. We all need at least one starch per day, so a baked sweet potato will more than cover that. Take a peek at its anti-inflammatory rating!

In the beginning, I included 1-2 scoops of Dave Draper's Bomber Blend protein and a scoop of milled flax seed. This witch's brew had an algae-looking film on top. So horrible looking, I named it "pond scum." I suffered the gag reflex with every gulp! After removing the two ingredients I just mentioned, the solution was nice 'n liquidy. Not all that bad, now.

But, for those of you who like eating these vegetables, you may love the blenderized version. It certainly is convenient and the body loves it. My wife, Janel, loves those vegetables, but cannot block out the initial appearance of "pond scum."

If I can do this, so can you.

It's kind of fun to do the impossible.
-Walt Disney

Glycemic Load

The **glycemic load (GL)** of each food is a number that estimates how much and how fast that food will raise a person's blood glucose level and how quickly the body will use it up. The GL accounts for how much carbohydrate is in the food, excluding fiber.

Originally, the **glycemic index (GI)** was invented in 1981 by Dr. Thomas Wolever and Dr. David Jenkins at the University of Toronto. It measured how quickly a carbohydrate food would raise the blood-glucose level. It did not take into account just how much of a carbohydrate food was fiber. Some carbohydrate foods are mostly fiber in content, so the actual blood-glucose levels were not that much an effect on blood-glucose. For example, watermelon has a high glycemic index number of 72, but with its higher fiber content, its GL rating is a low 3.6; not much sugar (glucose impact).

This is where the **glycemic load**, developed by Harvard researchers, became the standard.

GL Ratings
10 & Below - Good
11-19 - Acceptable
20 & Above – Avoid

You will discover all the foods from the anti-inflammatory list, with few exceptions, will fall in the "good" range, and none in the "avoid" range. But keep in mind, even amongst the pro-inflammatory foods, it's the processed and packaged foods that are the worst offenders.

If you are a diabetic, obese, or just want to lose weight, stay in the 10 and below range. When your blood glucose spikes high and quickly, it tumbles quickly, actually falling below the level prior to eating that food. With the lower glucose level, you get hungry again and eat. Can we say that obesity begins with these foods? With the lower GL number, the body takes longer to process a food into glucose, thereby utilizing it longer. This enables a more steady glucose level causing less desire to eat.

> You must be fit to give before
> you can be fit to receive.
> -James Stephens

ANTI-INFLAMMATORY FOODS (GOOD GUYS)

"IF" RATINGS

- Beef
- Pork
- Fish
- Ham
- Duck
- Bison
- Rabbit
- Deer
- Elk
- Lamb
- Cheese

- Fruits
- Fruit Juices
- Nuts
- Non-Starchy Vegetables
- Starchy Vegetables
- Cereals & Flour
- Peppers
- Chili Peppers
- Spreads
- Seasonings/Roots/Sweeteners
- Oils

IF Rating Scale
1 to 100 ... Mildly Anti-Inflammatory
100 to 500 ... Moderately Anti-Inflammatory
501 & Over ... Strongly Anti-Inflammatory

BEEF
IF ONLY (3 Oz)

	IF		IF
Arm Pot Roast		**Inside Skirt Steak**	
Braised	31	Broiled	25
Raw	11		
		Tip Round	
Blade Roast		Raw	17
Braised	27	Roasted	21
Raw	10		
		Ground	
Bottom Round		70% Lean Baked	3
Raw	17	Broiled	1
Roasted	10	Browned	3
Brisket		**Flanked Steak**	
Flat Half Raw	4	Raw	8
Braised	29	Broiled	10
Point Half Raw	19		
Braised	23	**Grass-Fed**	
Whole Raw	8	Ground Raw	4
Braised	15	Strip Steaks Raw	24
Tri-Tip Roast		**Rib**	
Raw	5	Large End Raw	3
Roasted	10	Broiled	2
		Roasted	17
Eye of Round		Small End Raw	6
Raw	23	Broiled	2
Roasted	23	Roasted	23

Rump Steak	IF	Top Loin Steak	IF
Grilled	13	Raw	12
		Broiled	7
Shoulder Roast			
Roasted	26	**Top Blade Steak**	
		Grilled	10
Shoulder Stead			
		Top Blade Roast	
Braised	8	Broiled	27
Tenderloin		**Corned Beef Brisket**	
Raw	8	Cooked	47
Broiled	8	Raw	39
Top Round Steak			
Raw	24		
Broiled	27		
Top Sirloin Steak			
Raw	16		
Broiled	13		

PORK
IF ONLY (3 Oz)

	IF
Tenderloin	
Broiled	9
Loin	
Whole Braised	6
Polish Sausage	
Pork	19
Pork Smoked	17
Canadian Bacon	
Grilled	3
Pork Bologna	
3 oz.	17

ALL FISH
IF ONLY (3 Oz)

Fish	IF	Octopus	IF
Grouper (Baked)	85	Raw	67
Bass (Fresh Water Raw)	133	Steamed	143
Bass (Fresh Water Baked)	169		
Bass (Striped Baked)	422	**Anchovy**	
Bass (Striped Raw)	329	Canned in oil-drained	871
Bluefish (Baked)	439	Raw	595
Bluefish (Raw)	343		
Caviar (Black & Red)	2,204	**Perch**	
		Baked	89
Catfish		Raw	70
Breaded & Fried	43		
Farmed & Baked	10	**Clams**	
Farmed & Raw	8	Breaded-Fried	45
Wild & Baked	38	Canned-Drained	82
Wild & Raw	32	Raw	44
		Steamed	166
Cisco (Raw)	106		
Cisco (Smoked)	448	**Crab**	
		Cakes	137
Cod		Blue (Canned)	87
Atlantic (Baked)	69	Blue (Raw)	114
Atlantic (Canned)	69	Blue (Steamed)	87
Atlantic (Dried & Salted)	225	Dungeness (Raw)	158
Atlantic (Raw)	80	Dungeness (Steamed)	204
Pacific (Baked)	78		
Pacific (Raw)	64	**Crayfish**	
		Farmed (Raw)	43
		Farmed (Steamed)	43

	IF		IF
Wild (Raw)	52	**Fish Oil (1 Tbsp)**	
Wild (Steamed)	58	Cod Liver	1061
		Herring	688
Croaker		Menhaden	1240
Atlantic (Breaded-Fried)	11	Salmon	1944
Atlantic (Raw)	40	Sardine	1107
Cutterfish		**Halibut**	
Raw	56	Baked	124
Steamed	125	Greenland (Baked)	497
		Greenland (Raw)	388
Drum		Raw	102
Freshwater (Baked)	48		
Freshwater (Raw)	38	**Herring**	
King (Raw)	60	Atlantic (Baked)	796
Steamed	197	Atlantic (Kippered)	855
Queen (Raw)	169	Atlantic (Pickled)	641
Steamed	212	Atlantic (Raw)	624
		Pacific (Baked)	814
White Fish		Pacific (Raw)	638
Smoked	96		
Baked	422	**Lobster**	
Raw	330	Northern (Raw)	102
		Northern (Steamed)	117
Whiting		Spiny (Raw)	49
Baked	222	Spiny (Steamed)	67
Raw	51		
		Mackerel	
Fish Sticks		Atlantic (Baked)	510
Frozen	61	Atlantic (Raw)	810
		Canned & Drained	465
		King (Baked)	214

	IF		IF
King (Raw)	169	**Rockfish**	
Pacific & Jack (Baked)	683	Pacific (Baked)	177
Pacific & Jack (Raw)	534	Pacific (Raw)	147
Salted	1663		
Spanish (Baked)	395	**Roe**	
Spanish (Raw)	414	Baked	1040
		Raw	813
Mullet			
Striped (Baked)	83	**Sablefish**	
Striped (Raw)	75	Baked	681
		Raw	532
Ocean Perch		Smoked	702
Baked	123		
Raw	102	**Salmon**	
		Atlantic (Farmed & Baked)	848
Oysters		Raw	725
Canned	254	Wild & Baked	489
Eastern (Breaded & Fried)	246	Wild & Raw	383
Eastern (Farmed & Baked)	271	Chinook (Baked)	582
Eastern (Wild & Baked)	290	Raw	689
Eastern (Wild & Raw)	220	Smoked	210
Eastern (Wild & Steamed)	345	Chum (Baked)	330
Pacific (Raw)	332	Canned & Drained	444
Pacific Steamed)	673	Coho (Farmed & Baked)	454
		Raw	421
Pollock		Wild & Baked	439
Atlantic (Baked)	223	Wild & Raw	354
Atlantic (Raw)	174	Wild & Steamed	446
Walleye (Baked)	210	Pink (Baked)	268
Walleye (Raw)	74	Canned	407
		Canned & Drained	442
		Raw	223

	IF		IF
Sockeye (Baked)	493	**Snapper**	
Canned & Drained	516	Baked	129
Raw	415	Raw	113
Sardines		**Rainbow Smelt**	
Atlantic (oil,drained)	435	Baked	334
Pacific (Tomato sauce-drained)	344	Raw	261
Scallops		**Squid**	
Bay & Sea (Steamed)	61	Fried	216
Breaded & Fried)	42	Raw	201
Raw	30		
		Sturgeon	
Sea Bass		Baked	107
Baked	344	Raw	84
Raw	262	Smoked	58
Sea Trout		**White Sucker**	
Baked	14	Baked	152
Raw	11	Raw	118
Shark		**Swordfish**	
Batter-dipped & Fried	201	Baked	349
Raw	276	Raw	293
Shrimp		**Tilapia**	
Breaded & Fried	28	Baked	63
Canned	219	Raw	50
Raw	35		
Steamed	76	**Tilefish**	
		Baked	274
		Raw	145

	IF
Trout	
Baked	209
Raw	164
Flounder	
Baked or Grilled	204
Rainbow Trout	
Farmed (Baked)	332
Farmed (Raw)	279
Wild (Baked)	308
Wild (Raw)	161
Tuna	
Bluefin Baked	593
Bluefin Raw	464
White in water	344
White in oil-drained	131
Yellowfin Baked	111
Yellowfin Raw	93
Light in oil-drained	106
Light in water-drained	110

HAM
IF ONLY (3 OZ)

	IF
Ham	
Canned	29
Slice Extra Lean	2
Steak	32
Ham & Cheese Loaf	16

DUCK
IF ONLY (3 OZ)

	IF
Meat Roasted	17
Meat & Skin Roasted	26
Meat & Skin Raw	31

BISON
IF ONLY (3 OZ)

	IF
Ground	
Cooked	2
Raw	19
Ribeye	
Broiled	21
Raw	27
Shoulder Roast	
Raw	25
Roasted	33
Top Round	
Broiled	23
Raw	26
Top Sirloin	
Broiled	22
Raw	29

RABBIT
IF ONLY (3 OZ)

	IF
Wild	
Raw	4
Stewed	22

DEER
IF ONLY (3 0Z)

	IF
Tenderloin Broiled	1
Top Round Broiled	2

ELK
IF ONLY (3 OZ)

	IF
Round Broiled	5

LAMB
IF ONLY (3 OZ)

	IF
Domestic Foreshank Braised	3
Quarters Cooked	175

CHEESE
(1 Cup)

	IF	GL
Non-Fat Swiss	20	4
Fat Free Mozzarella	20	2
Fat Free Mozzarella (Shredded)	20	2

FRUITS
IF (1/2 Cup) GL (1 Cup)

	IF	GL		IF	GL
Apricots			**Strawberries**		
Fresh	2	6	Fresh	14	3
Mango			Frozen		
Fresh	4	8	(unsweetened)	8	4
Kiwi					
Fresh	17	8	**Acerola Cherries**		
Blackberries			Fresh	342	1
Fresh	4	4	Fresh In juice	817	2
Cantaloupe			**Cherries**		
Fresh	37	5	Sour Fresh	6	
Orange			Sweet Fresh	7	
Fresh	5	5			
W/Peel	3	8	**Lemon**		
Pineapple			Peel Fresh 1 Tbsp	2	
Fresh	32	6	Fresh w/o Peel	9	4
Raspberries			Fresh w/Peel	14	3
Fresh	0	3	**Lime**		
Red/Pink Grapefruit			Fresh	3	1
Fresh	9	7			
White Grapefruit					
Fresh	1	5			

FRUIT JUICES

	IF	GL
Orange Juice		
Fresh 1/2 cup	1	9 (1 Cup)
Orange Drink Canned	13	6
V-8 Splash (8 oz.)		
Berry Blend	14	2
Diet Berry Blend	26	0
Diet Fruit Medley	26	0
Diet Strawberry Kiwi	26	0
Diet Tropical Blend	26	0
Tropical Blend	14	2
V-8 Fusion (8 oz.)		
Acai	5	5
Lemon Juice		
Juice Bottled		
(1/2 Cup)	8	1
Lemon Juice Fresh		
(1/2 Cup)	17	3
Lemonade From		
Mix 8 oz.	2	1
Sugar Free from		
Mix 8 oz.	3	0
Lime Juice		
Juice Bottled		
(1/2 Cup)	2	1
Fresh Juice (1/2 Cup)	7	3
Pineapple-Grapefruit		
8 oz	0	7
Carrot Juice		
Canned (1 Cup)	212	8

NUTS

	IF	GL		IF	GL
Almonds (1 Cup)			**Pistachios (1 Cup)**		
Raw	64	0	Dry-Roasted	16	4
Blanched	71	0	Raw	19	5
Dry-Roasted	66	0			
Honey Roasted	71	0	**Peanuts (1 Cup)**		
Oil-Roasted	77	0	Dry-Roasted	27	0
			Oil-Roasted	25	0
Cashews			Raw	20	0
Raw (1 Oz)	20	3			
Dry-Roasted (1 Cup)	27	15	**Flaxseed (1 Cup)**		
Oil-Roasted (1 Cup)	25	11	Fresh	39	0
Brazil Nuts			**Sunflower Seeds (1 Cup)**		
Raw	170		Raw	12	0
Macadamia (1 Cup)			**Hickory Nuts**		
Dry-Roasted	159	0	Raw (1 Cup)	30	
Raw	155	0	**Mixed Nuts (1 Cup)**		
			Dry-Roasted	61	1
Pecans			Oil-Roasted	37	0
Dry-Roasted (1 Oz)	65	0	Oil-Roasted/		
Oil-Roasted (1Cup)	45	0	No Peanuts	177	0
Raw (1 Cup)	46	0	Trail Mix w/Chocolate		
			Chips, Salted Nuts	33	

NON-STARCHY VEGETABLES
IF (1/2 Cup) GL (1 Cup)

	IF	GL		IF	GL
Broccoli			**Kale**		
Cooked	60	8	Cooked	112	3
Frozen/Cooked			Raw	0	3
Chopped	39	3	Frozen/Cooked		
Raw	26	3	(10 Oz)	213	4
Brussels Sprouts			**Beet Greens (1 Cup)**		
Cooked	40	5	Cooked	136	4
Raw	30	3	Raw	63	0
Asparagus			**Lettuce (1 Leaf)**		
Canned	34	3	Bibb	36	1
Cooked	38	2	Green Leaf	42	0
Raw	21	3	Iceberg	6	1
			Romaine	10	0
Spinach			Red Leaf	34	0
Canned	241	2			
Cooked	224	2	**Tomato**		
Raw	74	0	Cooked (Red Ripe)	9	4
Frozen/Cooked	187	2	Raw (Red Ripe)	9	2
			Green Raw	5	4
Cucumber			Sundried Oil	12	9
Peeled	1	1			
Raw	0	1	**Turnip Greens**		
			Cooked	238	1
Dandelion Greens (1 Cup)			Raw	134	1
Cooked	131	3			
Raw	150	2	**Watercress**		
			Raw	32	0

	IF	GL
Zucchini		
Cooked	14	1
Frozen/Cooked (10 Oz)	2	3
Raw	0	
Onions		
Cooked	240	8
Frozen/Cooked (10 Oz)	301	0
Raw	292	5
Sweet Raw	299	3
Okra		
Cooked	10	6
Frozen/Cooked (10 Oz)	15	6
Raw	9	3
Radish		
Oriental Cooked	2	1
Oriental Raw	5	3
Raw	4	1
Rhubarb		
Fresh	1	2
Frozen	3	1
Frozen/Cooked (1 Cup)	29	
Cabbage (1 Cup)		
Chinese Cooked	57	1

	IF	GL
Raw	30	1
Green Cooked	23	2
Raw	10	2
Red Cooked	3	1
Raw	12	2
Savoy Cooked	0	3
Raw	13	2
Cauliflower		
Cooked	9	1
Raw	13	2
Frozen/Cooked	12	1
Green/Cooked	11	2
Raw	9	2
Celery (1 Cup)		
Cooked	9	2
Raw	7	1
Collards		
Cooked	159	4
Frozen/Cooked (1 cup)	45	5
Raw (1 cup)	62	1
Green Beans		
Canned	3	3
Cooked	1	4
Frozen/Cooked (10 Oz)	1	3

	IF	GL
Mustard Greens		
Cooked (1 Cup)	172	0
Frozen/Cooked		
(10 Oz)	59	1
Swiss Chard		
Cooked	121	4
Raw (1 cup)	88	1
Mushrooms		
Brown	6	1
Portabella	1	2
Portabella Grilled	0	3
Parsley		
Dried (1 Tsp)	2	0
Fresh (1 Tbsp)	20	2 (1 Cup)
Sauerkraut		
Canned	4	2

STARCHY VEGETABLES
IF (1/2 Cup) GL (1 Cup)

	IF	GL		IF	GL
Pumpkin			**Winter Squash**		
Canned	168	6	Raw	4	
Cooked	49	3	Cooked	58	8
Raw	49	3			
			Butternut		
Carrots			Raw		
Canned (1 Tbsp)	79	0	Cooked	139	
Cooked (1 Tbsp)	130	0			
Frozen/Cooked			**Sweet Potato**		
(10 Oz)	90	2	Baked	189	10
Raw (1 Cup			Canned	45	24
Chopped)	98	3	Raw	76	11
Baby Raw (1 Large)	78	0			
			Green Peas		
Summer Squash			Frozen/Cooked		
Raw	20	2	(10 Oz)	9	13
Cooked	9	3			

CEREALS
IF (1 Cup) GL (1 Cup)

	IF	GL
General Mills		
Total	43	14
Kelloggs		
All Bran Extra Fiber	4	12
All Bran Buds	50	6
Bran Flakes	9	13

FLOUR

		IF	GL
Baker's Yeast			
Compressed			
(1 Pc)		27	1 (1 Cake)
Dry (1 Tsp)		19	1 (1 Tbsp)

PEPPERS

	IF	GL
Black Ground		
(1/2 Tsp)	1	
Cayenne (1/2 Tsp)	254	0
Green Cooked		
(1/2 Cup)	25	3
Frozen	11	0
Raw	24	2
Sauteed	43	0
Red Cooked	87	3
Frozen	32	2
Raw	39	3
Sauteed	61	1
White Ground		
(1/2 Tsp)	2	
Yellow Raw		
(1/2 Cup)	52	4

CHILI PEPPERS
IF (1/2 Cup) GL (1 Cup)

	IF	GL
Banana (Raw)	654	2
Hot (Raw)	1,024	2
Hot (Sun Dried)	1,366	8
Hungarian (Raw)	659	1
Jalapeno (Canned)	479	2
Jalapeno (Raw)	825	2
Serrano (Raw)	1,556	3
Green (Canned)	551	2
Hot (Canned)	701	2

SPREADS
IF (Varies)

	IF	GL
Almond Butter		
1/4 Cup	100	0
Peanut Butter (2 Tbsp)		
Crunchy	18	0
Smooth	10	0
W/Omega 3	91	0
Sunflower Seed Butter		
1/4 Cup	252	1
Cashew Butter		
1/4 Cup	72	1
Smart Balance		
Omega Plus	33	
Smart Balance Regular	5	
Mayonnaise (1 Tbsp)		
Olive Oil Light	34	
Smart Balance Omega		
Plus	15	
Mustard (1 Tsp)		
Prepared	2	5
Ground 1/2 Tsp	4	

SEASONINGS/ROOTS/SWEENERS

	IF	GL		IF	GL
Ginger			**Thyme**		
Root (1 Tbsp)	387	0	Dried (1 Tsp)	3	0
Ground (1/2 Tsp)	348	2	Fresh (1 Tbsp)	3	0
Pimento			**Taro**		
Canned (1/2 Cup)	54	3	Leaves Cooked		
			(1/2 Cup)	7	3
Sage			Raw (1 Cup)	31	1
Ground (1/2 Tsp)	1	0	Shoots Cooked		
			(1/2 Cup)	2	2
Salt			Raw	1	1
(1/2 Tsp)	0	0			
			Curry		
Spearmint			(1 Tsp)	116	1
Dried or Fresh	0	0			
			Flaxseed		
Garlic			(1/4 Cup)	26	0
Raw (1 Tbsp)	215	22 (1 Cup)			
Powder (1/2 Tsp)	468	3 (1 Tbsp)			
Turmeric					
(1/2 Tsp)	338	2			

OILS
IF (1 Tbsp) GL (1 Cup)

	IF	GL
Almond	64	0
Apricot Kernel	34	0
Avocado	68	0
Canola	80	0
Corn & Canola Blend	56	0
Enova	1	0
Flaxseed	13	0
Hazelnut	87	0
Olive	74	0
Safflower High Oleic	79	0
Sunflower High Oleic	101	0
Sardine	1107	0

PRO-INFLAMMATORY FOODS (BAD GUYS)

- Fruits
- Fruit Juices
- Nuts
- Non-Starchy Vegetables
- Starchy Vegetables
- Beans (Member of Starch Group)
- Rice (Member of Starch Group)
- Noodles/Spaghetti (Member of Starch Group)
- Beef
- Chicken/Duck
- Eggs
- Pork
- Ham
- Deer
- Elk/Moose
- Lamb
- Turkey
- Veal
- Hot Dogs
- Milk & Cottage Cheese
- Cheese
- Yogurt
- Cereals (Hot & Cold)
- Flour
- Bread
- Rolls & Biscuits2
- Muffins
- Crackers
- Spreads
- Dressings
- Seasonings/Roots/Sweeteners
- Desserts
- Coconut
- Granola
- Oils
- Poor Fast Food Choices

IF Rating Scale
-1 to -100 – Mildly Inflammatory
-101 to -500 – Moderately Inflammatory
-500 & Over – Strongly Inflammatory

FRUITS
IF (1/2 Cup) GL (1 Cup)

	IF	GL
Blueberries		
Fresh	-15	6
Frozen Unsweetened	-8	4
Frozen Sweetened	-34	16
Heavy Syrup	-70	20
Syrup Drained	-65	19
Dried Sweetened	-120	
Wild Frozen	-3	1
Blackberries		
Frozen	-12	6
Heavy Syrup	-65	22
Raw		4
Boysenberries		
Frozen	-4	4
Heavy Syrup	-65	21
Banana		
Fresh	-38	18
Chips-Dried (1oz)	-132	23
Apple		
Peeled	-10	3
With Skin	-9	3
Dried 1/4 cup	-49	26
Applesauce		
sweetened	-41	15
Applesauce		

	IF	GL
unsweetened	-15	5
Peaches		
Fresh (1 Large)	-10	5
Dried 1/4 cup	-76	46
Frozen sweet	-28	22
Heavy Syrup	-54	17
In Juice	-22	8
Light Syrup	-30	10
Syrup-Drained	-39	14
Pineapple		
Frozen Sweet	-64	19
Heavy Syrup	-56	19
In Juice	-36	12
Juice-Drained	-25	8
Light Syrup	-26	9
Plums		
Fresh	-10	5
Heavy Syrup	-70	21
In Juice	-25	12
Light Syrup	-38	12
Syrup-Drained	-49	15
Raisins		
Golden 1/4 cup	-136	75
Seedless 1/4 cup	-135	75

	IF	GL		IF	GL
Tangerines			**Raspberries**		
In Juice	-1	7	Frozen Sweet	-64	22
Light Syrup	-29	13	Heavy Syrup	-65	21
Drained	-3	5			
			Prunes		
Pears (1 Fruit)			Dried 1/4 cup	-91	54
Anjou Green Fresh	-16	5	Stewed	-82	25
Red Fresh	-12	5	Stewed w/sugar	-114	31
Asian Fresh	-7	2	In Juice	-51	16
Bartlett Fresh	-14	5			
Bosc Fresh	-16	5	**Watermelon**		
Dried 1/4 cup	-114	63	Fresh	-3	3
Heavy Syrup	-49	14			
In Juice	-26	7	**Strawberries**		
Light Syrup	-31	9	Frozen Sweet	-23	17
Syrup Drained	-36	10			
			Grapefruit		
Cherries			Canned in Juice	-6	7
Frozen Sweet	-76	22	Canned in Light		
Maraschino	-122	1	Syrup	-33	13
Sour Fresh	-3	6			
Sour Frozen	-9	5	**Grapes**		
Sour Heavy Syrup	-71	23	Red or White		
Sour In Juice	-8	6	(Green	-30	1
Sour Light Syrup	-63	18			
Sweet Fresh	-26	7	**Papaya**		
Sweet Heavy Syrup	-64	19	Heavy Syrup Drained		
Sweet In Juice	-38	11	1/2 cup	-215	20
Sweet Light Syrup	-45	14	In Juice Sweetened	-21	
Sweet Syrup Drained	-43	13	Fresh Juice	-9	9
Tart Dried-Sweet	-143				

	IF	**GL**
Cranberries		
Dried-Sweetened		
(1/4 cup)	-98	17 (1/3 Cup)
Fresh	-2	2

FRUIT JUICE
IF (1/2 Cup) GL (1 Cup)

	IF	GL		IF	GL
V-8 Splash Smoothies (8 Oz)			**Orange/Pineapple**		
Peach Mango	-37	2	1/2 cup	-11	13
Strawberry/Banana	-40	2			
Tropical Colada	-40	9	**Apple Juice**		
			1/2 cup	-12	6
Lemon Juice From Concentrate					
8 Oz	-33	2	**Grape Juice**		
Flavored Drink Mix			Pure	-30	12
(8 oz)	-5	11	Juice Canned	-34	12
Lemon-Lime Soda			Drink Canned	-40	10
(8 oz)	-36	1			
			Limeaide From Concentrate		
Grapefruit Juice			8 oz	-56	1
Juice (1/2 cup)	-7	7			
Fresh Juice (1/2 cup)	-3	7	**Orange Juice Drink**		
Sweetened	-17	9	Canned (8 oz)	-46	5
Prune Juice			**Passion Fruit**		
1/2 Cup	-51	16	Purple Juice Fresh	-7	9
			Yellow Juice Fresh	-24	13
Pineapple/Orange Juice			Fresh	-18	2
8 oz	-63	13			

NUTS
(1/4 Cup)

	IF	GL
Walnuts		
Black Raw	-35	0
English Raw	-34	0
Sunflower Seeds		
Dry-Roasted	-48	1
Oil-Roasted	-63	0
Sesame Seeds		
Hulled	-9	0
Unhulled	-5	0
Chestnuts		
Raw	-50	
Japanese		5
Chinese		7
European		7
Boiled	-36	
Japanese		1
Chinese		5
European		4
Roasted	-70	
Japanese		8
Chinese		9
European		42
Peanuts		
Boiled	-5	0

NON-STARCHY VEGETABLES
IF (1/2 Cup) GL (1 Cup)

	IF	GL		IF	GL
Eggplant			**Mushrooms**		
Cooked	-5	2	Brown Canned	-9	1
Raw	-2	1	Enoki Raw	-4	0
			Maitke Raw	-5	2
Beets			Oyster Raw	-5	5
Canned	-6	3	Shitake Cooked	-5	7
Cooked	-9	3	Straw Canned	-2	4
Raw	-1	5	White Raw	-3	2
Harvard Canned	-47		Portabella Raw	-3	2
Pickled	-34				
			Tomato		
Yellow Beans			Sundried (1/4 cup)	-16	12
Canned	-2	1	Canned Crushed	-12	1
Cooked	-3	4	Canned in Sauce	-2	6
			Canned Stewed	-9	6
Rutabagas					
Cooked	-4	5			
Raw	-3	4			

STARCHY VEGETABLES
(1/2 Cup)

	IF	GL		IF	GL
Pumpkin			Canned	-31	9
Pre-Mix Canned	-64	6	Raw	-32	2
Pie Spice (1 Tbsp)	-2	1	Mashed	-69	16
Seed Kernels Dried			Instant-Mashed	-52	98
(1/4 Cup)	-68	2	Hash Browned	-93	6
Seeds (Whole Roasted			Red Baked	-42	26
(1/4 Cup)	-28	22	Raw	-32	2
Corn			**Black-eyed Peas**		
On the Cobb	-111	6	Canned w/Pork		
Canned	-36	8	(1 cup)	-86	
Cooked	-76	17	Dried	-78	
Cream Canned	-56	18	Dried-Cooked (1 cup)	-19	
Frozen	-42	6			
Raw	-58	11	**Green Peas**		
Cornbread (1 oz)	-79		Canned	-4	4
			Cooked	-3	9
Potato					
White Baked	-47	13	**French Fries**		
Baked w/o Skin	-40	6	Frozen/Oven Baked	-51	8
Boiled w/o Skin	-44	26			

BEANS: (MEMBERS OF THE STARCH GROUP IF (1 Cup) GL (1 Cup)

	IF	GL		IF	GL
Kidney Beans			**Refried Beans**		
Canned (1 cup)	-66	15	Canned-Fat Free		
Dried-Cooked	-60	15	(1 Cup)	-74	12
Sprouted, Cooked,					
Boiled	-6	1	**Soy Beans**		
			Cooked	-13	
Lentils			Dried-Cooked		
Cooked/Boiled	-15	13	(1 Cup)	-44	
			Dry-Roasted (1 Cup)	-72	
Lima Beans			Roasted (1 Cup)	-83	
Canned		14			
Cooked	-45	14	**Fava Beans**		
Frozen/Cooked	-52	8	Canned (1 Cup)	-71	13
Large Dried Cooked			Raw	-34	10
(1 Cup)	-61	14	Dried-Cooked	-54	13
Raw	-29	48			
Small Dried Cooked	-48	16	**Great Northern Beans**		
			Canned (1 Cup)	-111	22
Navy Beans			Raw	-72	46
Canned (1 cup)	-108	21	Dried-Cooked		
Cooked (1 Cup)	-51	15	(1 Cup)	-55	13
Sprouted, Cooked,					
Boiled		1	**Black Beans**		
			Raw	-115	57
Pinto Beans			Dried-Cooked	-47	14
Canned (1 Cup)	-87	14			
Dried-Cooked			**Black Turtle Beans**		
(1 Cup)	-43	15	Canned (1 Cup)	-60	13
			Raw	-118	41

	IF	**GL**
Dried-Cooked	-80	19

Cow Peas

	IF	GL
Cooked	-14	
Dried	-69	
Dried-Cooked (1 Cup)	-54	
Frozen	-29	
Raw	-12	

Garbanzo (Chickpeas)

	IF	GL
Canned (1 Cup)	-82	23
Dried	-83	52
Dried-Cooked (1 Cup)	-70	17

Parsnips

	IF	GL
Raw	-8	7
Cooked, Boiled	-86	4

Baked Beans

	IF	GL
Baked Beans	-65	
w/Pork	-52	

RICE

	IF	GL
Brown		
Long Grain-Cooked		
(1 Cup)	-143	22
Medium Grain-Cooked		
(1 Cup)	-162	22
White		
Glutinous-Cooked		
(1 Cup)	-125	18
Long Grain-Cooked		
(1 Cup)	-153	22
Instant Cooked		
(1 Cup)	-131	
Medium Grain-Cooked		
(1 Cup)	-184	29
Short Grain-Cooked		
(1 Cup)	-188	30

NOODLES

	IF	GL
Chow Mein		
1 oz	-91	15 (1 Cup)
Egg (1 Cup)		
Cooked	-102	21
Rice (1 Cup)		
Cooked	-150	20
Spinach		
1 Cup	-56	

SPAGHETTI

	IF	GL
White Cooked		
(1 Cup)	-124	23
Spinach Cooked		
(1 Cup)	-120	20
Whole Wheat Cooked		
(1 Cup)	-82	15

BEEF
IF RATINGS ONLY (3 Oz)

Tongue

Raw	-265
Simmered	-17

Liver

Braised	-233
Pan Fried	-143
Raw	-8

Kidney

Simmered	-230
Raw	-70

Heart

Simmered	-168
Raw	-103

Porterhouse Steak

Broiled	-13
Raw	-11

Rib Eye

Broiled	-5

T-Bone Steak

Broiled	-18
Raw	-13

Tenderloin

Roasted	-8

Top Round Roast

Broiled	-1

Tripe

Raw	-26
Simmered	-53

Ground

70% Lean Raw	-6
80% Lean Raw	-5
Browned	-1
Broiled	-4
Baked	-4
90% Lean Raw	-6
Browned	-10
Broiled	-8
Baked	-7
95% Lean Raw	-6
Browned	-16
Broiled	-9
Baked	-4

Filet Mignon

Broiled	-26

Rump Steak

Raw	-9

Shoulder Medallion

| Raw | -10 |
| Grilled | -6 |

Top Blade Steak

| Raw | -5 |

CHICKEN
IF RATINGS ONLY (3 Oz)

Chicken Breast

Batter Fried	-48
Fried	-43
Raw	-19
Roasted	-25
Stewed	-24

Chicken Thigh

Batter Fried	-76
Fried	-89
Raw	-84
Roasted	-56
Stewed	-69

Chicken Wings

Batter Fried	-80
Fried	-93
Raw	-48
Roasted	-56
Stewed	-72

Chicken Leg

Batter Fried	-73
Fried	-79
Raw	-82
Roasted	-50
Stewed	-67

Chicken Heart

Raw	-604

Simmered	-502

Chicken Gizzard

Raw	-47
Simmered	-50

Giblets

Fried	-259
Simmered	-152

Liver

Pate Canned	-5
Pan Fried	-272
Raw	-138
Simmered	-274

Drumstick

Batter Fried	-70
Fried	-74
Raw	-78
Roasted	-59
Stewed	-58

Dark Meat

Fried w/o Skin	-97
Raw w/o Skin	-50
Roasted w/o Skin	-78
Stewed w/o Skin	-71

Light Meat

Fried w/o Skin	-57
Raw w/o Skin	-24
Roasted w/o Skin	-33
Stewed w/o Skin	-27

Cornish Hens

Roasted	-128
Roasted w/o Skin	-115
Raw	-106
Raw w/o Skin	-102

DUCK
IF RATINGS ONLY (3 Oz)

Duckling Roasted	-31
Duck Liver Raw	-29

EGGS
IF RATINGS ONLY (2 Oz)

Chicken Egg

White	-2
Whole	-85
Yolk	-182
Turkey Egg	-56
Quail Egg	-55
Goose Egg	-126
Duck Egg	-147

PORK
IF RATINGS ONLY (3 Oz)

Chops

Center Rib (Boneless)

Braised	-12
Broiled	-1
Raw	-45

Center Rib

Braised	-54
Broiled	-30
Pan Fried	-58
Raw	-18

Sirloin

Braised	-51
Broiled	-45
Raw	-14

Top Loin (Boneless)

Braised	-14
Broiled	-18
Pan Fried	-24
Raw	-16

Ground Pork

72% Lean

Cooked	-68
Raw	-62

96% Lean

Cooked	-49
Raw	-35
Extra Lean Crumbles	-14

Lean

Cooked	-49

Crumbles	-47
Raw	-52

Hocks

Pickled	-32

Loin

Whole Broiled	-2
Raw	-36
Roasted	-17

Ribs

Country Style

Braised	-40
Raw	-16
Roasted	-46
Raw	-48
Roasted	-52

Spareribs

Braised	-52
Raw	-474
Roasted	-64

Tenderloin

Raw	-20
Roasted	-16
Peppercorn Flavored	-17
Teriyaki Flavored	-20

Bacon

Grease (1 Tbsp)	-3
Raw	-90
Baked	-67
Microwaved	-91
Canadian-Uncooked	-29
Bacon Pan Fried	-36
Turkey Bacon	-206

HAM
IF RATINGS ONLY (3 Oz)

Country Style	-78
Honey Smoked	-16
Spiral Cut Roasted	-32
Turkey	-59
Water Added	-34

DEER
IF RATINGS ONLY (3 Oz)

Ground

		Shoulder Roast	
Browned	-60	Braised	-5
Raw	-49		

Loin

Broiled	-4
Raw	-69
Roasted	-99

ELK
IF RATINGS ONLY (3 Oz)

Ground Browned	-50
Ground Raw	-50
Loin Broiled	-7
Raw	-65
Roasted	-77

MOOSE
IF RATINGS ONLY (3 Oz)

Raw	-45
Roasted	-50

LAMB
IF RATINGS ONLY (3 Oz)

Domestic Leg

Raw	-18
Roasted	-15

Domestic Foreshank

Raw	-5

Domestic Loin

Broiled	-29
Raw	-43
Roasted	-43

Domestic Rib

Broiled	-77
Raw	-73
Roasted	-53

Domestic Shoulder

Braised	-51
Broiled	-31
Raw	-44
Roasted	-43

Ground

Broiled	-23
Raw	-49

TURKEY
IF RATINGS ONLY (3 Oz)

Neck

Simmered w/o Skin	-54
Raw w/o Skin	-48

Breast

Deli-Sliced	-12
Raw	-54
Roasted	-104

Dark Meat

Raw w/o Skin	-6
Roasted w/o Skin	-41

Giblets

Raw	-121
Simmered	-136

Gizzard

Raw	-49
Simmered	-43

Ground

Cooked	-80
Raw	-63

Heart

Raw	-153
Simmered	-201

Leg

Raw	-98
Roasted	-162

Liver

Raw	-123
Simmered	-184

Light Meat

Raw w/o Skin	-2
Roasted w/o Skin	-8

Smoked Turkey

3 Oz	-136

Wing

Raw	-54
Roasted	-103

VEAL
IF RATINGS ONLY (3 Oz)

Breast

Boneless Braised	-42
Boneless Raw	-33

Ground

Broiled	-56
Raw	-45

Kidneys

Braised	-114
Raw	-56

Leg

Braised	-44
Pan Fried Breaded	-63
Pan Fried Not Breaded	-38
Raw	-26
Roasted	-32

Liver

Braised	-138
Pan Fried	-160
Raw	-132

Loin

Braised	-92
Raw	-56
Roasted	-71

Rib

Braised	-63
Raw	-75
Roasted	-42

Shank

Braised	-42
Raw	-42

Shoulder Arm

Braised	-39

Shoulder

Braised	-53
Raw	-40
Roasted	-64

Sirloin

Braised	-63
Raw	-37
Roasted	-52

HOT DOGS
IF RATINGS ONLY (3 Oz)

Chicken	-47
Pork	-18
Turkey	-48

MILK & COTTAGE CHEESE

	IF	GL
Buttermilk Whole		
(1 Cup)	-76	9
Chocolate (1 Cup)		
Reduced Fat 2%	-114	14
Whole	-109	13
Low Fat 1%	-109	13
Condensed Sweetened		
(2 Tbsp)	-98	100
Evaporated (1/2 Cup)		
Fat Free	-48	15 (1 Oz)
Whole	-70	2 (1 Oz)
Milk (1 Cup)		
Fat Free	-52	9
Low Fat - 1%	-60	9
Reduced Fat - 2%	-71	9
Whole	-74	9
Goat Milk		
(1 Cup)	**-92**	**8**
Indian Buffalo	**-127**	**9 (1 Cup)**
Sheep Milk	**-122**	**9 (1 Cup)**
Chocolate Milkshake	**-183**	**3 (1 Oz)**

Vanilla Milkshake	-159	2 (1 Oz)
Soy Milk Chocolate **Light**	-67	21 (12 Oz)
Soy Milk Plain **Light**	-37	12 (12 Oz)
Soy Milk Vanilla **Light**	-47	17 (12 Oz)
Cottage Cheese (1/2 Cup)		
Creamed	-24	4 (4 Oz)
Fat Free	-23	6 (1 Cup)
Low Fat - 1%	-17	6 (1 Cup)
Reduced Fat - 2%	-21	7 (1 Cup)
Creamed w/Fruit	-24	8 (1 Cup)

CHEESE

Of all the 62 kinds of cheese currently on the market, all are on the **inflammatory** side of the scale with the exception of:

Non-Fat Swiss
Fat Free Mozzarella
Fat Free Mozzarella Shredded

The 59 other forms of cheese have an average inflammatory rating of **-32**, with whole milk **ricotta** measuring a robust **-62.**

This section not only includes each one's GL rating, but more importantly with this product, included are fat grams and calories. The findings will set you back on your heels.

CHEESE

	GL	Calories	Total Fat Grams
Mozzarella	2 (1 Cup)	336	25
Nonfat	2 (1 Cup)	168	0
Low Fat	1 (1 Cup)	413	29
Low Sodium	4 (1 Cup)	370	23
Parmesan			
Shredded	0 (1 Tbsp)	21	1
Hard	0 (1 Cubic Inch)	0	3
Low Sodium	2 (1 Cup)	456	30
Grated	2 (1 Cup)	431	29
American			
Pasteurized Lowfat	5 (1 Cup)	252	10
Pasteurized w/diSodium Phosphate	1 (Cup)	525	44
Pasteurized wo/di Sodium Phosphate	0 (1 Cubic Inch)	67	6
Swiss Cheese (Processed)			
Low Fat	5 (1 Cup)	238	7
Pasteurized w/di Sodium Phosphate	3	468	35
Pasteurized wo/di Sodium Phosphate	0	60	5
Swiss (Non-Processed)		502	37
Low Fat	3 (1 Cup)	236	7
Low Sodium	3 (1 Cup)	496	36
Blue Cheese	0 (1 Cubic Inch)	60	5
Cheddar	1 (1 Cup)	532	44
Low Fat	3 (1 Cup)	228	9

	GL	Calories	Total Fat Grams
Low Sodium	1 (1 Cup)	525	43
Colby	1 (1 Cup)	520	42
Low Fat	3 (1 Cup)	228	9
Low Sodium	1 (1 Cup)	525	43
Cheshire	1 (1 Oz)	108	9
Feta	4 (1 Cup)	396	32
Goat (Hard Type)	0 (1 Oz)	127	10
Semi-Soft	0 (1 Oz)	102	8
Soft	0 (1 Oz)	75	6
Limburger	0 (1 Cup)	438	37
Mexican Cheese			
Queso Anejo	3 (1 Cup)	492	40
Queso Asadero	2 (1 Cup)	470	37
Queso Chihuahua	3 (1 Cup)	494	39
Monterey	1 (1 Cup)	492	40
Low Fat	1 (1 Cup)	413	29
Cheese Fondue	7 (1 Cup)	492	29
Cheese Roquefort	1 (1 Pack)	324	26
American Cheese Food			
Pasteurized Process w/ Di Phosphate	8 (1 Pack)	745	56
Pasteurized Process w/o Di Phosphate	4 (1 Cup)	373	28
Nachos w/Cheese, Beans, Beef, Peppers	30 (6-8 Nachos)	569	31
Kraft Velveeta			
Pasteurized Process	1 (Oz)	85	6
Reduced Fat	2 (1 Oz)	62	3

	GL	Calories	Total Fat Grams
Sargento Ultra Thin			
Colby Jack	1 (3 Slices)	120	10
Cheddar	1 (3 Slices)	130	10
Borden Sharp Cheddar			
2% Milk	1 (1 Oz)	80	6
Provolone	2 (1 Cup)	463	35
Reduced Fat	1 (1 Slice)	77	5
Ricotta	7 (1 Cup)	428	32
Part Skim Milk	9 (1 Cup)	339	19
Romano	3 (5 Oz)	549	38
Cottage Cheese (1 Cup)			
(Large or Small Curd)			
Creamed	4	111	5
Creamed w/Fruit	8	219	9
1% Milk Fat	6	163	2
2% Milk Fat	7	194	6
Non-fat	6	104	0
Cream Cheese	2 (1 Cup)	794	79
Low Fat	11 (1 Cup)	482	37
Non-fat	1 (1 Oz)	39	0

YOGURT
(1 Cup)

	IF	GL
Fat Free Chocolate	-167	3
Fat Free Fruit	-145	21
Fat Free Plain	-56	11
Fat Free Vanilla	-60	1
Greek Berry (Chobani)	-108	
Low Fat Fruit	-151	23
Low Fat Low Sugar	-150	21
Low Fat Plain	-66	10
Lot Fat Vanilla	-107	17
Soy	-125	11
Whole Milk Plain	-72	8
Frozen Yogurt Chocolate	-66	19
Frozen Yogurt Fat Free, Sugar Free	-43	19

CEREALS
IF (1 Cup) GL (1 Cup)

	IF	GL		IF	GL
Health Valley			**Nabisco**		
Oat Bran Flakes	-115	12	Cream of Rice		
Fiber 7 Flake	-110	13	Regular prepared	-78	11
Quaker			**General Mills**		
Oat Bran	-43	1	Oatmeal Crisp		
Oat Bran Raw	-24	12	w/Almonds	-196	28
Oatmeal Squares	-104	27	Oatmeal Crisp w/		
Oatmeal Squares w/			Apple Cinnamon	-177	30
Cinnamon	-110	29	Oatmeal Crisp		
Oatmeal Instant			w/Raisin	-224	32
Flavored Prepared	-106	11	Wheaties	-43	13
Oatmeal Instant			Wheaties Raisin Bran	-136	27
Prepared	-62	13	Cheerios	-27	12
Oatmeal Regular			Cheerios Apple		
Prepared	-84	13	Cinnamon	-86	17
Oats Whole Grain			Cheerios Frosted	-68	16
(1/3 Cup)	-137		Cheerios Honey Nut	-62	13
Life	-64	16	Cheerios Multi-Grain	-51	15
			Cheerios Yogurt		
Life Cinnamon	-28	16	Burst	-82	16
Cream of Wheat			Corn Chex	-73	18
Flavored Prepared	-136	14	Corn Chex Frosted	-121	20
Cream of Wheat			Chex Honey Nut	-147	20
Instant Prepared	-75	15	Chex Multi-Grain	-69	23
Cream of Wheat			Chex Rice	-55	17
Regular Prepared	-78	13	Chex Wheat	-95	23
			Cinnamon Grahams	-129	18
			Cinnamon Toast		

	IF	GL
Crunch	-91	16
Cinnamon Toast Crunch Reduced Sugar	-72	
Cookie Crisp	-83	18
Fiber One (1/2 Cup)	-11	6
Honey Nut Clusters	-190	31
Golden Grahams	-116	18

Kellogg's

	IF	GL
Rice Krispies	-71	20
Raisin Bran	-143	12
Raisin Bran Crunch	-190	
Raisin Nut Bran	-191	26
Cocoa Krispies	-152	19
Cocoa Pebbles	-150	
Corn Flakes	-96	17
Corn Flakes Honey Crunch	-145	18
Corn Flakes Reduced Sodium	-141	17
Corn Pops	-102	20
Fruit Loops	-90	
Fruit Loops Reduced Sugar	-71	19
Frosted Flakes	-151	20
Frosted Flakes Reduced Sugar	-128	20
Frosted Rice Krispies	-152	20
Fruit Harvest w/Berries	-125	17
Honey Smacks	-123	17

	IF	GL
Apple Jacks	-90	21
Crispix	-65	18
Crispy Brown Rice	-130	18
Cracklin' Oak Bran	-147	19
Coco Pops		20
Mini-Wheats Frosted w/Strawberries		29
Special K	-34	14
All Bran		8

Post

	IF	GL
Shredded Wheat (1 Cup)	-156	26
Shredded Wheat n'Bran Spoon size	-188	24
Shredded Wheat Honey Nut	-157	
Grape Nuts (1/2 Cup)	-152	16
Honey Bunches of Oats	-74	17
Honey Bunches of Oats Honey Roasted	-91	16
Honeycombs	-119	18
Alpha Bits	-64	18
Alpha Bits w/Marshmallows	-118	18
Fruity Pebbles	-138	17
Golden Crisp	-117	8
Banana Nut Crunch	-121	27

Malt-O-Meal (Instant)
(1 Cup – all GL)

	IF
Puffed Rice	10
Puffed Wheat	7
Puffed Raisin Bran	25
High Fiber Bran Flakes	13
Blueberry Muffin Tops	16
Cinnamon Toasters	15
Apple Cinnamon	16
Frosted Flakes	20
Honey Nut Toasty O's	16
Golden Puffs	24
Cocoa Dyno Bites	19

FLOUR
IF (1/3 Cup) GL (1 Cup)

	IF	GL
Rice		
Brown	-198	81
White	-220	91
Oat		
1/3 Cup	-103	11 (1 Oz)
Soy		
Full Fat	-23	11
Low Fat	-7	9
Sesame Seed		
1/3 Cup	-68	3 (1 Oz)
Corn Flour		
Degermed	-186	77 (1 Cup)
Masa White	-132	
Masa White Enriched	-119	51
Masa Yellow Enriched	-118	61
White Whole Grain	-135	56
Yellow Whole Grain	-134	56
Cornmeal		
Degermed White	-198	88
Degermed Yellow	-197	88
Self-Rising White	-146	78
Self-Rising Yellow	-146	78
Whole Grain White	-140	58
Whole Grain Yellow	-139	58

	IF	GL
Corn Starch	-216	
Buckwheat		
Flour	-100	44
Barley		
Flour	-139	62
Malt Flour	-173	78
Hulled	-140	65
Pearled Cooked		
(1 Cup)	-127	19
Pearled Raw	-175	80
White Flour		
All Purposed Bleached	-141	66
All Purpose Self-Rising	-134	64
All Purpose Unbleached	-141	66
Flour Bread	-142	68
Flour Cake	-174	76
Whole Wheat		
Flour	-89	44
Peanut Flour		
Defatted	-1	6
Potato Flour		
Defatted		88

BREAD
IF (1 Slice) GL (1 Slice)

	IF	GL
Multi-Grain	-34	5
Oatmeal	-40	7
Reduced Calorie	-50	7
Banana	-70	19
Oat Bran	-32	6
Reduced Calorie	-22	6
Raisin	-47	9
Pumpernickel	-40	6
Pita (Whole Wheat)	-47	17
Italian	-49	9
Rye	-41	8
Reduced Calorie	-19	3
Rice Bran	-34	6
Cracked Wheat	-42	1
Bread Sticks Plain	-80	21
Bread Crumbs	-91	51
Sourdough	-261	
Wheat	-49	5
Bran	-39	9
White	-53	14
Whole Wheat	-38	5
Reduced Calorie	-22	
Wheat Germ	-47	8
Croutons	-84	14

French Toast

	IF	GL
Frozen	-38	10
Homemade	-30	9

ROLLS & BUSCUITS
IF (1 Oz) GL (1 Roll or Biscuit)

	IF	GL
Cinnamon	-70	24
Egg Roll	-49	11
French	-48	11
Hamburger		
(Low Calorie)	-26	7
Hot Dog		
(Low Calorie)	-26	7
Hamburger		
(Multi-Grain)	-33	10
Hot Dog		
(Multi-Grain)	-33	10
Hamburger (White)	-55	13
Hot Dog (White)	-55	13
Kaiser	-56	18
Oat Bran	-32	7
Pumpernickel	-51	10
Rye	-51	13
Wheat	-39	7
White		
(Brown & Serve)	-61	26
Whole Wheat	-44	11
Biscuits from Mix	-61	8
Multi-Grain	-54	
Refrigerated Dough	-62	14
Reduced Fat	-60	

MUFFINS
IF (1 Oz) GL (1 Muffin)

	IF	GL
Blueberry	-75	10
Blueberry Low Fat	-59	13
Corn	-63	5
Corn From Mix	-53	8
Oat Bran	-48	4
English Muffin Cinnamon Raisin	-48	16
English Muffin Mixed Grain	-43	17
English Muffin Plain	-53	16
English Muffin Wheat	-39	13
English Muffin Whole Wheat	-26	12

CRACKERS
IF (1 Oz) GL (Varies)

	IF	GL
Ritz	-94	6 (5 Crackers)
Low Sodium	-77	
Cheese Filling	-64	6
Peanut Butter Filling	-56	5
Rye	-60	20 (1 Cup)
Crispbread	-81	24 (1 Cup)
Cheese Filling	-58	5 (1/2 Oz)
Saltine	-106	3 (2 Crackers)
Fat Free	-114	9 (3 Crackers
Reduced Fat	-95	
Wheat w/cheese	-67	6 (1/2 Oz)
w/Peanut Butter	-54	5 (1/2 Oz)
Triscuit	-78	33 (1 Cup)
Reduced Fat	-88	
Wheat Thins	-88	33 (1 Cup)
Low Sodium	-59	33 (1 Cup)
Cheese Crackers	-89	14 (6 Crac.)
w/Peanut butter	-52	13 (6 Crac.)
Matzo Plain	-119	17 (1 Crac.)
White Wheat	-67	11 (1 Crac.)
Egg & Onion	-101	14 (1 Crac.)
Egg	-114	15 (1 Crac.)

	IF	GL
Melba Toast	-91	15 (1 Cup)
Rye &		
Pumpernickel	-90	7 (1/2 Oz)
Wheat	-80	7 (1/2 Oz)

SPREADS

	IF	GL
Butter (1 Tbsp)		
Light	-25	0 (1 Oz)
Salted	-44	0 (1 Cup)
Unsalted	-44	0 (1 Cup)
Whipped	-24	0 (1 Cup)
Margarine (1 Tbsp)		
Butter Blend	-17	0 (1 Tbsp)
Stick Reduced		
Fat	-10	0 (1 Tbsp)
Tub Reduced		
Fat	-5	0 (1 Tbsp)
Sesame Seed Butter		
Tahini		
1/4 Cup	-20	0 (1 Tbsp)
Mayonnaise (1 Tbsp)		
Light	-13	11 (1 Cup)
Soybean & Saf-		
flower Oil	-60	0 (1 Cup)
Soybean Oil		
(Hellman's)	-37	0 (1 Cup)
Tofu	-11	2 (1 Cup)
Cholesterol		
Free	-33	1 (1 Cup)
Honey		
1 Tbsp	-78	169 (1 Cup)

	IF	GL
Maple Syrup		
1 Tbsp	-58	126 (1 Cup)
Molasses		
1 Tbsp	-69	155 (1 Cup)
Peanut Butter (2 Tbsp)		
Reduced Fat	-21	4 (1 Oz)
Cream Cheese (1 Oz)		
Regular	-48	2 (1 Cup)
Fat Free	-7	1 (1 Oz)
Reduced Fat	-30	11 (1 Cup)

DRESSINGS
IF (2 Tbsp) GL (1 Cup)

	IF	GL		IF	GL
Bacon Tomato	-22	0	Balsamic Vinegar		
Blue Cheese	-39	0	(1 Tbsp)	-7	
Fat Free	-24	29	Peppercorn	-52	
Light	-13	16	Poppyseed Creamy	-46	
Buttermilk Light	-20	1	Ranch	-41	0
Caesar	-42	0	Light	-19	1
Fat Free	-35		Russian	-41	32
Light	-16	16	Light	-27	30
Coleslaw	-38	22	Sesame	-36	0
Light	-36		Thousand Island	-26	9
French	-21	2	Fat Free	-25	34
Fat Free	-28	35	Light	-3	1 (2 Tbsp)
Light	-17	30			
Green Goddess	-27	0			
Honey Mustard	-36	4			
Honey Fat Free	-41				
Honey Light	-14				
Italian	-16	4			
Fat Free	-6	8			
Light	-8	2			
Oil & vinegar	-36				

SEASONINGS/ROOTS/SWEETNERS

	IF	GL
Persimmon		
Fresh 1/2 Cup		
(Native)	-19	4 (1 Fruit)
Fresh ½ Cup		
(Japanese)		8 (1 Fruit)
Dried 1/4 Cup	-51	11 (1 Fruit)
Soy Sauce (1 Tbsp)		
Shoyu	-3	11 (1 Cup)
Shoyu Low		
Sodium	-2	12 (1 Cup)
Tamari	-4	1 (1 Tbsp)
Soy Pasta		
Dried 1 Oz	-100	
Sugar		
Brown	-77	150 (1 Cup)
Granulated	-63	2 (1 Packet)
Powder	-42	84 (1 Cup)
Sucralose (Splenda)		
1 Packet	-4	1
Aspartame (Equal)		
1 Packet	-5	0
Tomato Paste/Sauce		
Paste 2 Tbsp	-4	9 (1 Cup)
Puree 1/2 Cup	-12	8 (1 Cup)

	IF	GL
Sauce 1/2 Cup	-6	6 (1 Cup)
Sauce w/Cheese		
1/2 Cup	-39	
w/Mushrooms		
1/2 Cup	-3	8 (1 Cup)

Tofu (1/2 Cup)
Soft	-17	2 (1 Slice)
Firm	-22	2 (1 Slice)
Silken Light Firm	-24	1 (1 Slice)

Cinnamon
Ground 1/2 Tsp	-1	1 (1 Tbsp)

DESSERTS
IF (1 Oz) GL (1 Piece)

	IF	GL
Danish (1 Oz)		
Cheese	-30	14
Cinnamon	-33	35
Fruit	-46	37
Lemon	-52	19
Nut	-34	16
Pie Crust (1 Oz)		
Chocolate Cookie	-55	72
Frozen	-46	58
Graham Cracker	-49	86
Refrigerated	-92	98
Vanilla Wafer	-54	11
Cream		
Half & Half		
(1 Tbsp)	-8	8 (1 Cup)
Fat Free	-5	1 (1 Oz)
Heavy	-18	0 (1 Cup)
Heavy Whipped		
2 Tbsp	-18	0 (1 Cup)
Light 1 Tbsp	-16	1 (1 Cup)
Table	-12	6
Liquid Light	-3	6
Powdered	-11	29
Powdered Light	-6	47 (1 Cup)

	IF	GL
Croissant (1 Oz)		
Apple	-46	11 (1 Med.)
Cheese	-61	11 (Small)
Plain (Butter)	-63	7
Pie (1 Oz)		
Apple	-36	21
Banana Cream	-39	208
Blueberry	-35	22
Boston Cream	-46	21
Cherry	-37	26
Chocolate Cream	-61	15
Chocolate Mousse/ Mix	-38	14
Coconut Cream	-41	12
Coconut Custard	-33	16
Dutch Apple	-44	34
Egg Custard	-24	10
Fried Cherry	-40	27 (1 Pie)
Fried Fruit	-39	27 (1 Pie)
Fried Lemon	-40	27 (1 Pie)
Lemon Meringue	-63	29
Mince	-54	44
Peach	-33	19
Pecan	-63	49
Pumpkin	-26	181
Vanilla Cream	-40	22

DESSERTS - COOKIES
IF (1 Oz) GL (1 Cookie)

	IF	GL
Chocolate Chip	-102	4
Reduced Fat	-99	5
Slice & Bake	-88	
Sandwich	-86	6
Extra Filling	-59	5
Wafer	-100	50 (1 Cup)
Devil's Food Fat Free	-105	11
Coconut Macaroon	-126	12
Brownie	-68	21
Animal Crackers	-92	36 (1 Box)
Fig Bars	-86	18
Fortune Cookie	-122	5
Frosted Lemon	-87	
Fruit & Honey	-96	
Ginger Snap	-99	4
Graham Cracker	-105	43 (1 Cup)
Chocolate Coated	-135	6
Hermit	-97	12
Lady Finger	-106	5
Marshmallow Chocolate		
Coated	-75	11
Molasses	-93	16
Oatmeal W/Raisins	-74	7
Oatmeal Slice &		
Bake	-73	5

	IF	GL
Peanut Butter	-64	5
Sandwich	-74	6
Slice & Bake	-72	5
Pecan Shortbread	-51	5
Raisin	-82	
Shortbread	-71	3
Sugar	-81	7
Sugar Wafer w/		
Cream Filling	-112	4
Slice & Bake	-75	6
Vanilla Wafer	-82	3
Reduced Fat	-99	38 (1 Cup)
Sandwich W/		
Cream Filling	-99	7
White Macadamia		
Nut		17

DESSERTS - ICE CREAM

	IF	GL
Ice Cream Bar (1 Bar)		
Chocolate Covered	-86	
Crunch Coating	-300	
Chocolate (1/2 Cup)	-83	8
Light	-78	9
Light Sugar Free	-90	9
Premium	-93	15
Soft Serve Chocolate	-99	11 (1/2 Cup)
Light	-86	
Vanilla	-79	8
Fat Free	-73	4
Light	-97	10
Light Sugar Free	-75	7
Premium	-158	12
Soft Serve	-99	11 (1/2 Cup)
Light	-73	9
Dairy Queen Cones		
Chocolate		20
Vanilla		19
Dipped Chocolate		22
Breyers (1/2 Cup) (GL Only)		
Chocolate 98% Fat Free		9
Vanilla 98% Fat Free		9
Light French Choc.		11

	IF	GL
Light French Vanilla		9
Light Mint Choc. Chip		10
Lig Vanilla Choc. Straw.		9
Vanilla Fudge Twirl (No Sugar)		9
Choc. Caramel (No Sugar)		9
Butter Pecan (No Sugar)		7

DESSERTS - DOUGHNUTS
IF (1 Oz) GL (1 Doughnut)

	IF	GL
Chocolate Sugar Glazed	-56	19
Cruller Sugar or Glazed	-65	15
Plain	-36	13
Chocolate Frosted	-73	5
Sugar or Glazed	-52	20
Wheat Sugar or Glazed	-45	6
Cream Filled	-16	13
Jelly Filled	-34	18
Raised Glazed	-62	

DESSERTS - CHOCOLATE

	IF	GL
Chocolate Soda (8 Oz)	-33	1 (1 Oz Carbonated beverage)
Baking Unsweetened (1 Oz)	-36	0 (1 Cup)
Dark Chocolate (1 Oz)	-77	13 (1 Bar)
Extra Dark (1 Oz)	-64	
70-85% Cocoa		15 (1Bar)
60-69% Cocoa		26 (1 Bar)
45-59% Cocoa		46 (1 Bar)
Milk (1 Oz)	-103	13 (1 Cup)
Semi-Sweet (1 Oz)	-81	47 (1 Cup)
Cocoa Powder Unsweetened (1 Tbsp)	-2	16 (3 Tsp)
Cocoa From Mix (8 Oz)	-93	2 (1 Oz)
Sugar Free From Mix (8 Oz)	-45	1 (1 Oz)
Chocolate Syrup		16 (2 Tbsp)

COCONUT
IF (Varies) GL (1 Cup)

	IF	GL
Milk Canned (1/2 Cup)	-239	5
Coconut Water (8 Oz)	-18	3
Coconut Dried (1/4 Cup)	-100	0 (1 Oz)
Dried-Sweetened (1/4 Cup)	-77	22
Dried-Toasted (1/4 Cup)	-104	6 (1 Oz)
Raw (1/4 Cup)	-56	1

GRANOLA
IF (1/2 Cup) GL (1/2 Cup)

	IF	GL
Homemade	-92	31
Kellogg's Low Fat		
w/o Raisins	-82	27
Low Fat w/Raisins	-96	31
Nature Valley Low Fat w/		
Fruit	-166	29
Quaker 100% Natural Low		
Fat w/Raisins	-90	29
Quaker Oats & Honey	-113	21
Sun Country w/Almonds	-113	23

Granola Bars (1 Bar)

Hard plain		9
Coconut/Chocolate		8
Hard Almond		9
Oats, Fruits, Nuts		14
Peanut Butter, Milk Choc.		10
Fruit Filled Non-Fat		13

OILS
IF (1 Tbsp) GL (1 Cup)

	IF	GL
Cocoa Butter	-40	0
Coconut	-115	0
Corn	-50	0
Cotton Seed	-94	0
Palm	-28	0
Palm Kernel	-99	0
Peanut	-3	0
Poppy Seed	-78	0
Rice Bran	-12	0
Safflower High Linoleic	-91	0
Sesame	-21	0
Soybean	-38	0
Sunflower Linoleic	-77	0
Walnut	-25	0
Wheat Germ	-54	0
Grapeseed	-87	0

POOR FAST FOOD CHOICES

IF Ratings Only

Pizza Hut (1 Pc)

Cheese-Stuffed Crust	-157
Pepperoni-Thin Crust	-137
Sausage-Classic Crust	-169
Sausage-Deep Dish	-190
Sausage-Thin Crust	-148

Domino's (1 Pc)

Sausage-Classic Crust	-169
Sausage-Deep Dish	-190
Sausage-Thin Crust	-114

1 Serving of the Following:

Applebee's Chicken Tender Platter	-303
Crunchy Onion Rings	-724
Burger King's Onion Rings	-350

Cracker Barrel's Onion Rings	-551
Fried Chicken Tenderloin Platter	-235
Denny's Chicken Strips	-277
Onion Rings	-357
Spaghetti & Meat-balls	-292
TGI Friday's Chicken Fingers	-302
Wendy's Crispy Chicken Sandwich	-216
Subway 6" Roast Beef on White Bread	-118

Fast Foods With Cheese

	GL	Calories	Fat Grams
Carl's Junior (1 Order)			
American Cheese	0	49	4
Salad Dressing Blue Cheese	0	320	35
Swiss Style Cheese	0	50	4
Potato, Bacon Cheese	35	640	29
Cheese Danish Dessert	27	400	23
Del Taco (1 Order)			
Egg, Cheese Burrito	18	450	24
Chili, Cheese Fries	23	670	46
Deluxe Chili, Cheese Fries24	710	49	
Hardee's (1 Order)			
1/3 Bacon, Cheese, Thick Burger	23	910	63
2/3 Bacon, Cheese, Thick Burger	24	1,300	96
Hot Ham'n Cheese Sandwich	14	287	13
Big Hot Ham'n Cheese Sandwich	20	435	20
Chili, Cheese Fries	31	700	39
Chick-Fil-A (1 Order)			
Bacon, Egg, Cheese Biscuit	20	470	26
Sausage, Egg, Cheese Biscuit	23	630	40
Egg, Cheese Biscuit	19	400	21
Chicken, Cheese Biscuit	23	470	23
Chicken, Egg, Cheese Bagel	24	500	20
Blue Cheese Dressing (1 Tbsp)	0	150	16

	GL	Calories	Fat Grams
Hot Pockets (1 Pkg)			
Ham'N Cheese	42	681	28
Little Caesar's Pizza (1 Slice)			
14" Cheese, Deep Dish	16	268	10
14" Cheese, Thin Crust	5	148	8
14" Cheese, Regular Crust	14	236	8
McDonald's (1 Order)			
Bacon, Egg, Cheese Biscuit	15	432	27
Double Quarter Pounder w/Cheese	18	760	48
Quarter Pounder w/Cheese	19	513	28
Ham, Egg, Cheese Bagel	30	550	23
Cheese Danish Dessert	25	400	21
Papa John's Pizza (1 Slice)			
14" Cheese Original Crust	20	304	11
14" Cheese Thin Crust	11	257	14
Cheese Dipping Sauce	1	70	6
Blue Cheese Dipping Sauce	0	170	18
Pizza Hut (1 Slice)			
14" Cheese Regular Crust	17	271	11
14" Thin Crust	11	225	10
Blue Cheese Dressing	0	140	14
Subway Sandwich (6") & Soup (1 Order)			
Steak & Cheese	22	390	14
Salad Steak & Cheese	8	180	8
Cheese & Egg	16	320	15

	GL	Calories	Fat Grams
Soup: Potato, Cheese Chowder	11	210	10
Broccoli & Cheese	4	180	12

Taco Bell (1 Order)

	GL	Calories	Fat Grams
Chili, Cheese Burrito	19	390	18
Chalupa Nacho Cheese Steak	12	340	21
Chalupa Nacho Cheese Chicken	12	340	20
Nacho Cheese Sauce	2	110	10
Cheese Quesadilla	18	490	29

Wendy's (1 Order)

	GL	Calories	Fat Grams
Jr. Hamburger w/Cheese	16	330	15
Hot Stuffed Baked Potato			
Bacon w/Cheese	37	580	22
Egg, Sausage, Cheese Biscuit	10	460	34

Blue Cheese Dressing

	GL	Calories	Fat Grams
Cheddar Cheese Shredded	0	260	27
(2 Tbsp)	0	70	6

Summary

Food measurements for counting calories uses weight in grams. The following three nutrients are most important:

> 1 Gram of a Carbohydrate = 4 calories
> 1 Gram of a Protein = 4 calories
> 1 Gram of a Fat or Alcohol = 9 calories

Basically, a carbohydrate is everything non-animal or fish. In terms of calories, the non-starchy vegetables contain but 20-25 calories per ½ cup yet require about 15-20 calories for digestion. Try to gain weight here. Whether pro-inflammatory or anti-inflammatory, these figures apply. Pro-inflammatory non-starchy vegetables also have an insignificant negative **IF** ratings. Starchy vegetables, whether pro-inflammatory or anti-inflammatory, carry approximately 70 calories, but the negative IF rating for pro-inflammatory starchy vegetables is quite significant.

So what's the answer? Eat non-starchy vegetables primarily from the anti-inflammatory list and trickle in some from the pro-inflammatory side. Starch is an important nutrient, so limit it to the anti-inflammatory side. That takes care of your vegetables. How hard can that be? No worry about counting calories, figuring portion sizes, and juggling the all-important inflammation issue.

For cooking oils, stay on the anti-inflammatory side; there are plenty! Those on the pro-inflammatory side are a huge risk for the most part.

Meats are mostly favorable in terms of **IF** rating, but stay away from animal organs. Beef is a good choice, but surprisingly, chicken needs to be accompanied by strictly anti-inflammatory vegetables, especially peppers and chili peppers. Chili peppers are off the chart anti-inflammatory. The difficult task comes from sifting through mainstream health articles and promotions.

I just received an article touting coconut oil for cooking. It has a long shelf-life and can resist creating high heat carcinogens; cancer promoters. It's even been shown to improve cognitive qualities of those with Alzheimer's disease. Believe me, it tastes good. However, its **IF** rating is -115; moderately high at one tablespoon. That single tablespoon might not be enough for cooking. Three tablespoons and your **IF** rating now equals -345. Toss in some beef liver and you have another -143; total now is -478. That's a big hole to climb out from. You probably will not be able to avoid finishing the meal on the pro-inflammation side.

The same beef liver at -143 fried in canola oil at +80, gives you a reasonable start of -63. Toss some cooked carrots on your plate at +130 and your result is a friendly +73. If you don't like cooked carrots, place a baked sweet potato on your plate at +189, and your result is a whopping +146.

Honey has been praised weekly in my email inbox for its wonderful qualities. One tablespoon of God's food is a -78. It has been pushed ferociously to replace all sweeteners. Besides the rather dreadful negative **IF** rating, its glycemic load (GL) indicator is off the chart at 169; anything over 20 is awful. Use judiciously. Sweeten your cereal with strawberries. I love honey, but I am "in love" with a healthy body, seeing how like everyone else, I get only one.

Too many "health practitioners" are only concerned with the outer body composition. If you are "roped in" to mainstream hysteria, you'll "hollow-out" yourself. But, you'll leave an attractive corpse for the viewing. Gimmicks do not work anywhere in life.

Anytime you read about or are told of a food's healthy qualities, check this book for its **IF** rating. A poor **IF** rating will trump the food's nutritious value. It's then time to find an alternative food with a positive **IF** rating.

An occasional delicious processed (boxed, packaged, etc.) food will make eating and living somewhat worthwhile. But if you live out of the box or package, there is no hope for you. At some point, that insistence on ignoring the inevitable reality will leave you with depressing deathbed regrets. All you can really hope for is listening resides on your "hard drive."

> Every man has a right to his opinion, but no
> man has a right to be wrong with his facts.
> -Bernard W. Baruch